APPLICATIONS MANUAL FOR

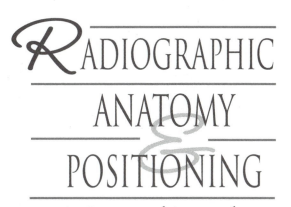

RADIOGRAPHIC
ANATOMY
& POSITIONING

An Integrated Approach

Diane H. Gronefeld, MEd, RT (R)
Associate Professor
Radiologic Technology Program
Department of Allied Health, Human Services, and Social Work
Northern Kentucky University
Highland Heights, Kentucky

Mary L. Madigan, RT (R) (M)
Clinical Coordinator
Radiologic Technology Program
Bellevue Community College
Bellevue, Washington

With Drawings by Carolyn Autenrieth, RT (R)

D0073794

Notice: The authors and the publisher of this volume have taken care to make certain that the doses of drugs and schedules of treatment are correct and compatible with the standards generally accepted at the time of publication. Nevertheless, as new information becomes available, changes in treatment and in the use of drugs become necessary. The reader is advised to carefully consult the instruction and information material included in the package insert of each drug or therapeutic agent before administration. This advice is especially important when using, administering, or recommending new and infrequently used drugs. The authors and publisher disclaim all responsibility for any liability, loss, injury, or damage incurred as a consequence, directly or indirectly, of the use and application of any of the contents of this volume.

98 99 00 01 02/ 10 9 8 7 6 5 4 3 2 1

Prentice Hall International (UK) Limited, *London*
Prentice Hall of Australia Pty. Limited, *Sydney*
Prentice Hall Canada, Inc., *Toronto*
Prentice Hall Hispanoamericana, S.A., *Mexico*
Prentice Hall of India Private Limited, *New Delhi*
Prentice Hall of Japan, Inc., *Tokyo*
Simon and Schuster Asia Pte. Ltd., *Singapore*
Editora Prentice Hall do Brasil Ltda., *Rio de Janeiro*
Prentice Hall, *Upper Saddle River, New Jersey*

Library of Congress Cataloging-in-Publication Data

Gronefeld, Diane H.
    Applications manual for Radiographic anatomy & positioning : an integrated approach / by Diane H. Gronefeld and Mary L. Madigan ; drawings by Carolyn Autenrieth.
        p.   cm.
    ISBN 0-8385-8247-8 (pbk. : alk. paper)
    1. Radiography, Medical—Positioning.   2. Radiography, Medical—Positioning—Atlases.   3. Radiography, Medical—Positioning—Examinations, questions, etc.   I. Madigan, Mary L.   II. Cornuelle, Andrea Gauthier Radiographic anatomy & positioning.   III. Title.
    [DNLM: 1. Radiography—methods—examination questions.
2. Posture.   WN 160 C819r 1997 Suppl.]
RC78.4.G76   1997
616.07′572′076—dc21
DNLM/DLC
for Library of Congress   96-48080
                                                        CIP

Acquisitions Editor: Kim Davies
Production Editor: Elizabeth Ryan
Designer: Janice Barsevich Bielawa

PRINTED IN THE UNITED STATES OF AMERICA

"The future belongs to those who believe in the beauty of their dreams."
Eleanor Roosevelt

TABLE OF CONTENTS

RATIONALE

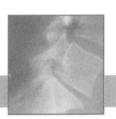

You will learn a substantial amount of information in the radiologic technology program that will enable you to become an excellent radiographer. Although everything you will learn is important, you must have a solid foundation in positioning and related anatomy before you can perform even the most basic radiographic procedures. The acquisition of information and building of this foundation will take place in many ways. You must first learn the most basic information and then add other, more in-depth facts. Once the whole picture is complete, you must be able to evaluate a given situation and determine the correct procedure. This Applications Manual is a valuable tool that will help you build a broad base of learning and understanding.

Basic anatomy and positioning is often learned through memorization and recall of detail, along with the repetition of doing basic radiographic exams. The first component of Chapters 2 through 12 consists of drawings that represent radiographic projections. Coloring and labeling the drawings will help you achieve an excellent comprehension of what is visualized on the various positions and projections, and reinforce how the exams should be performed. Each illustration is drawn in the correct orientation as it would be viewed on the viewbox, with a right or left marker appropriately placed. The worksheets that accompany the drawings include basic positions and projections of the chest, abdomen, and bony anatomy that you will need to know as a beginning radiographer.

The Study Question section of each chapter was specifically done in a "fill-in-the-blank" format to encourage you to look up the answer when necessary rather than guessing on a multiple choice answer. These questions are intended to reinforce your knowledge of basic anatomy and positioning as presented in the drawings, as well as introduce complex situations that require more thoughtful answers.

Acquiring basic positioning skills will allow you to radiograph patients under normal circumstances. Many times, however, unusual circumstances may prevent the radiographer from radiographing the patient in the optimal position as originally learned. In these instances, it is necessary to synthesize available information and decide on the best course of action before the exam can be successfully accomplished. In an effort to facilitate this kind of learning, case studies involving atypical patients are included in Chapter 2 through 18. These case studies are presented to encourage you to think about how you might adapt your knowledge of routine positioning to perform an exam under unusual circumstances. Students are often uncomfortable answering questions when there is no exact answer. With practice, however, you should be able to work your way through the case studies with a minimum of difficulty and maximum of creativity.

You have chosen an exciting, dynamic profession that demands the production of consistent, quality radiographs for optimal diagnoses. This Applications Manual will help you in your quest to become an excellent radiographer.

Diane H. Gronefeld, MEd, RT (R)
Mary L. Madigan, RT (R) (M)

OBJECTIVES

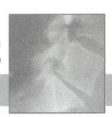

Upon successful completion of the units, the student will be able to:

1. Identify the basic anatomy of the chest and abdomen.
2. Name and describe the bones of the skeleton, and the articulations formed by adjoining bones.
3. Describe the basic anatomy and physiology of the respiratory, urinary, biliary, digestive, and cardiovascular systems, and the mammary glands.
4. Discuss routine radiographic examinations of the skeletal, respiratory, urinary, biliary, and digestive systems with regard to patient positioning, centering, and evaluation criteria.
5. Identify the structures best demonstrated on routine radiographic projections.
6. Discuss non-routine radiographic procedures that are performed to examine the cardiovascular system and mammary glands.
7. Define terminology associated with the positions/projections, to include anatomy, procedures, and pathology.
8. Briefly discuss how to achieve the positions/projections requested when circumstances dictate that the patient cannot be radiographed under normal conditions.
9. Describe how to work around an immobile or disabled patient to obtain the positions/projections requested, while maintaining the greatest patient comfort possible.
10. Develop problem-solving skills by studying situations involving atypical patients and working through them to achieve optimal radiographs under adverse conditions.
11. Develop an understanding of appropriate radiographs that should be obtained to visualize basic pathology.

DIRECTIONS

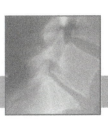

▶ POSITIONING WORKSHEETS

Each drawing represents a radiographic position or projection, with the anatomy presented as it would appear on the radiograph. Color the anatomy that is best demonstrated on each projection. Label the anatomy that is specified on the cover page for each chapter. Complete the appropriate information sheet for each drawing.

▶ STUDY QUESTIONS

Answer each of the questions with the best possible solution. The answers to most questions are very brief (one or two words), while some of the questions ask for longer explanations.

The answers to the study questions are provided in the *Instructor's Resource Manual* for the textbook, *Radiographic Anatomy & Positioning: An Integrated Approach.*

▶ CASE STUDIES

Write a specific explanation detailing how you would handle radiography of the patient in each case study. Describe as many details as possible in your description, including how the patient is positioned, type and placement of the cassette, centering landmark(s), central ray angulation, and appropriate patient care skills. When specific pathology is mentioned, explain how it will be visualized on the radiograph. Answer specific questions that may be included with the case studies.

While there is no exact solution for each of the case studies, some ideas and procedural considerations are identified in the *Instructor's Resource Manual* for the textbook, *Radiographic Anatomy & Positioning: An Integrated Approach.*

INTRODUCTION TO RADIOGRAPHY

► STUDY QUESTIONS

1. The set of ethical rules that members of the radiologic technology profession are expected to follow with regard to professional conduct and patient care are known as the_____ .

2. Briefly discuss how your personal attitudes can affect patient care. _____
   _____
   _____
   _____

3. A four-year-old child has been brought to the radiology department by her parents for a radiographic examination of the chest. Discuss the method of communication you will use to successfully complete the exam. _____
   _____
   _____
   _____

4. A radiographer sneezes several times while positioning an elderly inpatient for an examination. Three days later, the patient develops an upper respiratory infection. Explain why the patient's illness can be described as a nosocomial infection. _____
   _____
   _____

5. Following Universal Precautions, when should a radiographer wear a mask or a face shield? _____
   _____

6. You are working with another radiographer to complete a radiographic examination of the abdomen on a patient in strict isolation. Describe your role in the procedure as the "dirty" or contaminated radiographer. _____
   _____
   _____
   _____

7. _____ is a term that refers to the physical characteristics of the body, including shape, size, muscle tone, and position of internal organs.

8. Radiographs of the foot were ordered on a patient whose history indicated that he stepped on a metal wire, which was still in his foot. What is the minimum number of projections that should be taken by the radiographer? Explain your answer. _____
   _____

9. A patient having an average body habitus is described as _____ .

10. The _____ plane divides the patient into equal anterior and posterior portions.

11. A _____ plane divides the body into right and left sections.

12. The anterior or front aspect of the body is also referred to as the _____ surface.

13. If the direction of the central ray was described as *cephalic*, the x-ray beam would be directed _____ (away from/toward) the patient's head.

QUESTIONS 14–20: USE THE TERMS PROXIMAL, DISTAL, MEDIAL, OR LATERAL TO DESCRIBE THE FOLLOWING RELATIONSHIPS.

14. The wrist is _____ to the elbow.

15. The shoulder is _____ to the elbow.

16. The nose is _____ to the right eye.

17. The toes are _____ to the ankle.

18. The ankle is _____ to the knee.

19. The left ear is _____ to the eye.

20. According to anatomical position, the thumb is on the _____ side of the hand.

QUESTIONS 21–30: USE TERMS THAT REFER TO PART/BODY MOVEMENT TO COMPLETE EACH STATEMENT.

21. Turning the foot outward at the ankle joint is called _____ .

22. _____ refers to movement toward the midline of the body.

23. _____ is the decrease in the angle of a joint by bending.

24. _____ refers to straightening of a joint.

25. Turning the hand to place the palm down is known as _____ .

26. _____ refers to the circular movement of a structure around a specified axis.

27. The term _____ is often used in skull positioning to refer to a movement of the head in which the sagittal plane is not parallel to the long axis of the body and/or the table.

28. The act of turning on to one's back is known as _____ .

29. To abduct the leg, an individual must move the leg _____ (away from/toward) the midline of the body.

30. As you are ice skating, your ankles turn inward. This movement is called _____ .

QUESTIONS 31–38: USE POSITIONING/PROJECTION TERMINOLOGY TO COMPLETE EACH STATEMENT.

31. When your patient is lying on his left side, he is in a/an _____ position.

32. The term _____ describes a position in which the patient is rotated between lateral and the prone or supine position.

33. According to anatomical position, which surface of the hand faces forward? _____

34. The term _____ refers to the direction in which the central ray travels through the body.

35. When a patient is in a/an _____ position, she is lying flat on her back.

36. When the patient is in a/an _____ position, the head is positioned lower than the feet.

37. A/an _____ projection is one in which the central ray skims the structure to produce a profile projection.

38. Define *posteroanterior (PA)* as it relates to a projection.

_____

_____

QUESTIONS 39–43: IDENTIFY THE PROJECTIONS OR POSITIONS DESCRIBED IN THE FOLLOWING STATEMENTS.

39. The patient is lying on his back with the central ray passing horizontally from one side to the other. _____

_____

40. The patient is in a near lateral position with the top leg brought in front of the lower leg, which causes her to roll slightly toward a left anterior oblique position.

_____

41. The patient is lying on his abdomen, with the right anterior side of the body nearest the film. _____

_____

42. The patient is standing with her right posterior side away from the film and left posterior side closest to the film.

_____

43. Since your patient was having slight difficulty breathing in a recumbent position, you placed him in the _____ position by elevating his head approximately 45°.

44. What type of information may be included on the patient identification permanently stamped on the radiograph?

_____

_____

_____

45. Your patient is standing with his left side against the upright Bucky tray and his right side toward the x-ray tube. Which marker will you place on the cassette? Explain your answer. _____

_____

46. _____ refers to the overall blackening of the film and is controlled by the amount of radiation reaching the film.

47. What is "SID"? _____

_____

48. _____ controls the penetration of the radiation, while _____ controls the quantity of radiation produced.

49. The difference in density between two adjacent areas of a radiograph is known as _____ .

50. A radiograph of the hand was taken using low kVp. Since the resultant image is mostly black and white with few shades of gray, it can be described as having _____ (high/low) contrast.

51. The chest is an anatomical area that has _____ (high/low) subject contrast due to the differences in tissue densities.

52. As you position an elderly patient for a projection of the skull, you place a sponge under her head. The sponge elevates her head approximately 2 in. off of the table, thereby increasing OID. How does this affect magnification of the part?_____

_____

53. Prior to making an exposure, radiographic film is placed in a light-proof holder called a/an _____

_____

54. Where are intensifying screens located? _____

_____

55. The use of _____ (fast/slow) intensifying screens will result in greater sharpness and less radiographic density than _____ (fast/slow) screens.

56. A device composed of lead strips and placed between the patient and the x-ray tube to absorb scatter radiation is called a/an _____ .

57. How does the radiographer know which photocells to select when using automatic exposure control (AEC)?

_____

_____

58. What is the *ALARA* concept of radiation protection?

_____

_____

59. To facilitate patient positioning, a _____ tabletop will move freely in any direction with the release of a lock.

60. _____ equipment differs from a general radiographic room as it permits the observation of dynamic physiologic function. It is usually used for radiographic examinations of the gastrointestinal tract.

61. The _____ is a mobile unit that is capable of fluoroscopy and radiography. It is often used in surgery for pacemaker insertion and reduction of fractures.

62. A type of radiography that demonstrates anatomy by using motion to blur out structures above and below the area of interest is known as _____ .

63. The radiographer will use an instrument known as _____ to measure the thickness of a part prior to setting technical factors for a radiographic examination.

64. _____ are radiolucent positioning aids that can be used to cushion and support the patient during radiographic examinations.

65. When more than one exposure is being taken on a single cassette, masking can be used to block x-rays since it is made of _____ .

66. Exposure to radiation may mutate cells and cause _____ effects, which affect future generations.

67. Reducing the size of the x-ray field to film size or smaller is known as _____ .

68. The three primary rules of radiation protection are concerned with _____ , _____ , and _____ .

69. You just took a PA projection of the chest. Explain how the radiograph should be displayed on the viewbox. _____

_____

_____

_____

70. What do the abbreviations CT and MRI stand for? _____

_____

_____

71. _____ is a special tomographic technique that uses x-ray tubes, special radiation detectors, and a computer to produce sectional images of tissue.

72. An imaging modality that uses sound waves to differentiate between solid and fluid-filled structures is known as

_____ .

73. In place of ionizing radiation, MRI examinations use _____ waves in addition to the nuclei of the hydrogen atoms in the body and a strong magnetic field to construct images.

74. In nuclear medicine, a radiation-emitting material known as a/an _____ is administered to the patient, localized in a specific area of the body, and detected by a gamma camera.

75. List several devices that are used to monitor the amount of radiation received by an occupational radiation worker.

_____

_____

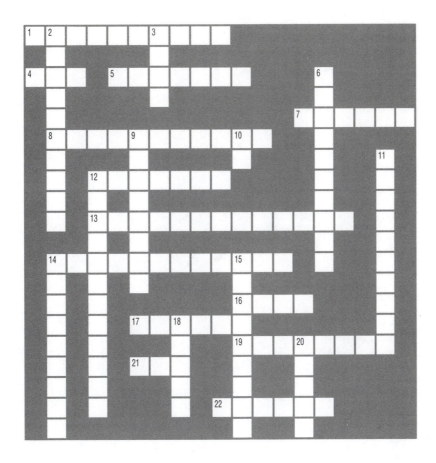

ACROSS

1. Central ray skims one point of the structure
4. Position in which left anterior side is closest to the film
5. Position in which the patient is rotated between lateral and AP or PA
7. Describes angulation of the CR toward the patient's feet
8. Plane that divides the body into equal right and left halves
12. Position in which the patient is rotated 90° from true AP or PA
13. The patient's head is tilted lower than the feet
14. Flexion movement between the lower leg and foot so that the angle between the two structures is less than or equal to 90°
16. Opposite of projection and is used when discussing the radiographic image
17. Patient is lying flat on his or her back
19. Describes the movement of the head when turning it from side to side (ie, when indicating "no")
21. Position in which patient's right posterior side is closest to the film
22. Refers to the posterior or back part of the body

DOWN

2. Upright position with head facing straight, arms down with palms forward
3. Misalignment of the body part so that the sagittal plane is not parallel with the rest of the body or the table
6. Plane dividing the body into upper and lower regions
9. Body habitus of a very thin person in which the thorax is narrow and shallow, diaphragm is very low, and heart is long and narrow
10. The CR passes from the posterior to the anterior aspect of the body
11. The direction in which the central ray travels through the body
12. Position in which the patient is lying on his or her side and the CR is directed horizontally to either the patient's front or back aspect
14. The patient is in a recumbent position and the CR is directed horizontally
15. Turning the foot inward at the ankle joint
18. Patient is lying on his or her abdomen in a face down position
20. The CR is angled longitudinally with the long axis of the body

COLOR THE HEART, LUNGS, AND BONY ANATOMY EACH A DIF-
FERENT COLOR AND LABEL THE FOLLOWING ANATOMICAL
PARTS ON THE DRAWINGS FOR THIS SECTION. LABEL ALL
PARTS THAT CAN BE SEEN ON EACH POSITION OR PROJEC-
TION.

CHEST: PA, Left Lateral, and Right Lateral Decubitus

► LUNGS	► TRACHEA	► BONY ANATOMY	► FUNDUS OF STOMACH
Apex	Carina	Scapulae	► DIAPHRAGM
Base	► LEFT AND RIGHT MAIN	Clavicles	
Hilum	STEM BRONCHI	Ribs	
Costophrenic angle	► HEART SHADOW	Vertebral column	

COMPLETE THE APPROPRIATE INFORMATION SHEET FOR
EACH DRAWING.

2

RESPIRATORY SYSTEM

► PA CHEST

CENTERING LANDMARK AND CR ORIENTATION

PATIENT POSITIONING

MAIN STRUCTURES VISUALIZED

NOTES

PA CHEST

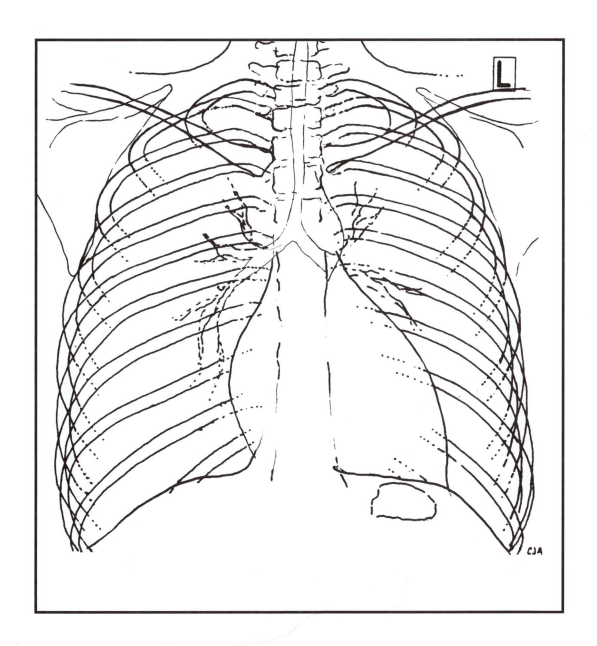

► LEFT LATERAL CHEST

CENTERING LANDMARK AND CR ORIENTATION

PATIENT POSITIONING

MAIN STRUCTURES VISUALIZED

NOTES

LEFT LATERAL CHEST

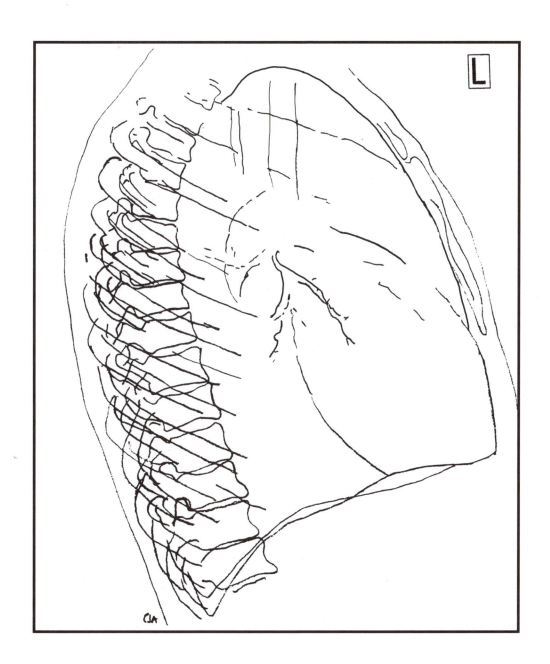

► RIGHT LATERAL DECUBITUS CHEST

CENTERING
LANDMARK AND CR
ORIENTATION

PATIENT
POSITIONING

MAIN STRUCTURES
VISUALIZED

NOTES

RIGHT LATERAL DECUBITUS CHEST

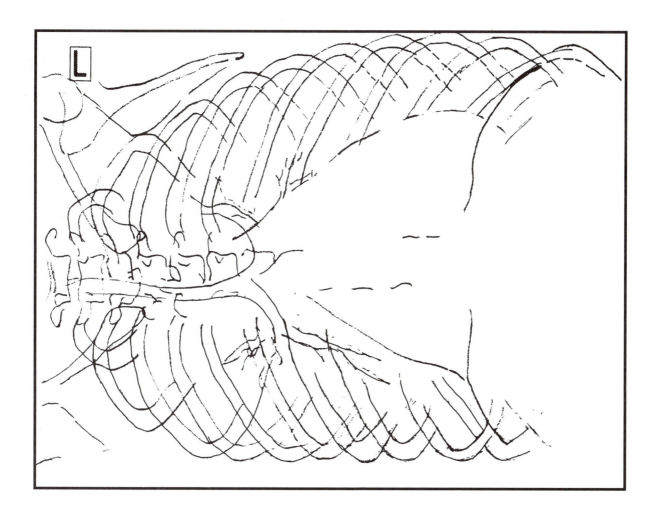

► STUDY QUESTIONS

1. The four main components of the respiratory system include:

   A. _____

   B. _____

   C. _____

   D. _____

2. A function of the mouth and nose is to _____ _____ the incoming air before it passes to the lungs.

3. The _____ , or throat, functions in both the respiratory and digestive systems.

4. The _____ is a leaf-shaped flap of cartilage that forms a lid over the laryngeal opening during swallowing.

5. The _____ bone is a small horseshoe-shaped bone located at the base of the tongue in the anterior neck.

6. The _____ is also known as the voice-box.

7. The division of the pharynx located behind the mouth is the _____ .

8. Tracheostomies are usually performed just below the ring of cartilage forming the inferior margin of the larynx and known as the _____ cartilage.

9. A prominent landmark in the neck corresponding to the level of the 5th cervical vertebra is the _____ _____ .

10. The trachea is approximately _____ in. (_____ cm) in length and is located _____ (anterior/posterior) to the esophagus.

11. What supports the trachea and continually keeps it open as a passageway for air? _____ _____

12. The trachea bifurcates at the level of _____ into the right and left _____ .

13. The _____ is a ridge of cartilage found at the lower end of the trachea at the point of bifurcation. It is used as a landmark for placement of ET tubes.

14. Why are inhaled foreign bodies more likely to pass into the right lung rather than the left lung? _____ _____ _____

15. The right primary bronchus branches into _____ smaller secondary bronchi, while the left primary bronchus branches into _____ smaller secondary bronchi.

16. What are bronchioles? _____ _____

17. The small clusters of small air sacs found at the terminal branching of the bronchioles are called _____ .

18. The upper rounded end of the lungs situated above the clavicles is called the _____ .

19. The exchange of O_2 and CO_2 takes place between the _____ and surrounding capillaries.

20. The concave, inferior surface of each lung is called the _____ .

21. The primary bronchi and pulmonary vessels enter the lungs at the area known as the _____ .

22. The _____ _____ of a lung is formed on the lateral aspect of the lung's lower margin where the ribs meet the diaphragm.

23. The right lung is divided in three lobes by the horizontal and oblique _____ .

24. The double fold of membrane covering the outer surface of the lungs is the _____ . Specifically, the _____ _____ lies adjacent to the lungs, while the _____ _____ is adjacent to the thoracic cavity.

25. Freshly oxygenated blood is transported from the lungs to the heart by the right and left _____ _____ .

26. The thoracic and abdominal cavities are separated from each other by the dome-shaped _____ .

27. The _____ is a spongy, elastic material that allows the lungs to expand and contract during respiration.

28. The space in the thoracic cavity between the lungs that is occupied by the heart, great vessels, trachea, esophagus, and thymus gland is called the _____ .

29. Very small blood vessels called _____ have permeable walls that allow for the transfer of O_2, CO_2, and some fluids.

30. On the average, a person will inhale and exhale approximately _____ times per minute.

31. What does the root word -*pnea* mean? Define *dyspnea.* _____ _____

32. When taking a patient's clinical history prior to chest radiography, why is it important to ask about previous thoracic surgery? _____ _____ _____

33. When a person inhales, his/her diaphragm moves _____ (superiorly/inferiorly).

34. Your patient did not roll her shoulder and arms forward on the PA projection of the chest. How is this positioning error obvious on the radiograph? _____ _____

35. On a good inspiratory PA projection of the chest, at least _____ posterior ribs should be demonstrated.

36. Why is it important that a patient elevate his/her chin for a PA projection of the chest? _____ _____

37. Asymmetry of the _____ on a PA projection of the chest indicates rotation.

38. When setting the technical factors for chest radiography, the radiographer should select _____ (low/high) kVp to adequately penetrate the heart and mediastinum.

39. Due to the tissue differences between the heart and the lungs, the chest is described as having _____ _____ subject contrast.

40. What is the normal range of kVp used in chest radiography? _____

41. If AEC is not employed and the technical factors are set manually, a time of 1/20 second or less is recommended for chest radiography. Explain why such a short time is important. _____ _____

42. The recommended SID for chest radiography is _____.

43. Which of the three AEC cells is/are selected for a lateral projection of the chest? _____ _____

44. What are the recommended breathing instructions for chest radiography? _____ _____

45. The ER physician asked for the *single best projection* that would demonstrate the epiglottis and upper trachea on an infant with suspected epiglottitis. What projection would you take? _____

46. Which lateral decubitus projection would best demonstrate the amount of pleural effusion present in the left lung? _____

47. Which lateral decubitus projection would best demonstrate a pneumothorax in the right lung? _____ _____

48. What area of the chest is best demonstrated on a lordotic projection? _____

49. Which projection of the respiratory system would demonstrate the following structures: the air-filled pharynx, larynx, and trachea superimposed over the spine? _____ _____

50. You have a requisition to take a lordotic projection of the chest on a patient who was transported to the radiology department by stretcher. He informs you that he must remain flat on his back due to a recent spinal injury. How will you modify the procedure to get an acceptable radiograph? _____

_____

_____

51. The heart will appear more magnified on a/an _____ _____ (AP/PA) projection.

52. A 3-month-old infant has been sent to the radiology department for radiographs of her chest. Since the AEC is not working correctly on your machine, you must manually set the technical factors. You have a good technique for an average-sized adult; how will you convert it to an acceptable technique for this child? _____

_____

53. Using the mobile unit, you must take an AP projection of the chest on a patient who is semi-erect in bed. She tells you that she cannot sit completely erect as she is in a great deal of pain. You decide that you must angle the central ray to compensate for her position. How will you determine the direction and degree of angulation? _____

_____

_____

54. Referring to the previous question, your efforts produced a radiograph that resembled a lordotic projection. When you repeat the radiograph, what change(s) will you make?

_____

_____

55. Some pathologies that are _____ (additive/destructive) in nature require a reduction in exposure factors.

FOR QUESTIONS 56–62, INDICATE WHICH OF THE FOLLOWING PATHOLOGIC CONDITIONS ARE ADDITIVE OR DESTRUCTIVE PROCESSES. A = ADDITIVE, D = DESTRUCTIVE

56. _____ pneumonia

57. _____ edema

58. _____ pneumothorax

59. _____ pleural effusion

60. _____ active tuberculosis

61. _____ bronchiectasis

62. _____ emphysema

63. On a PA projection of the chest, the central ray should be directed to the level of _____ .

64. As you are viewing a chest series that you just completed, you observe that the positioning on the lateral is "perfect." How do you make the determination that there is no rotation evident? _____

_____

65. When positioning for a/an _____ projection of the chest, the patient's mid-sagittal plane will be at a 45° angle to the film with the right anterior surface of his chest touching the chest unit.

66. Which side of the patient's chest would you place closest to the film for a lateral projection if the patient had a history of a previous myocardial infarction? _____

_____

67. What is the centering point for an AP projection of the upper airway? _____

_____

68. On a correctly rotated 45° right anterior oblique projection, the _____ side of the chest should appear approximately twice as wide as the opposite side.

69. On a lateral projection of the upper airway, the region from _____ to _____ should be visualized on the radiograph.

INDICATE TRUE OR FALSE FOR QUESTIONS 70–74.

_____ 70. A grid is usually not employed for chest radiography since the lungs are air-filled.

_____ 71. A poor inspiration on a PA chest radiograph may cause the heart to appear enlarged.

_____ 72. The esophagus should be visible in the medi-astinum on a PA projection of the chest.

_____ 73. Braided hair can create an artifact on a radiograph of the chest if it hangs in the collimated field.

_____ 74. To accurately demonstrate air–fluid levels in the lungs, a horizontal beam must be employed, even if the patient is in a semi-erect position.

75. Complete the following table:

Projection	CR Angle/Angle of Part	Centering Point	Film Size	Structures Seen
Lateral upper airway				
Left anterior oblique				
Right lateral decubitus				

▶ WORD SEARCH

USING THE FOLLOWING CLUES, FIND TERMI-NOLOGY RELATED TO THE RESPIRATORY SYS-TEM IN THE WORD SEARCH PUZZLE.

1. Dyspnea and wheezing caused by spasmodic constriction of the bronchial tree
2. Absence or cessation of respiration
3. Chronic obstructive pulmonary disease
4. Disease of the lungs characterized by inflamed lesions
5. Inflammation of the bronchi
6. Inflammation of the pleura
7. Condition in which the lungs appear overinflated because air is trapped in the alveoli, making respiration difficult
8. Inflammation of the lungs with congestion
9. Deprivation of oxygen to the body tissue and organs
10. Blood in the pleural cavity
11. Bluish coloration of the skin resulting from deficient oxy-genation
12. Whooping cough
13. Inhalation of a foreign material
14. Inflammation with swelling of the epiglottis
15. Collapsed lung

```
S  A  M  H  Y  C  E  S  D  C  A  Z  A  P  K
I  I  P  N  E  U  M  O  N  I  A  M  R  K  X
S  O  T  N  F  M  E  B  J  J  H  J  A  X  G
O  B  B  I  E  W  O  Y  T  T  W  E  H  F  F
L  Q  R  A  T  A  A  T  S  Q  H  Y  M  T  U
U  R  O  M  H  T  N  A  H  I  P  W  T  J  H
C  P  N  E  U  M  O  T  H  O  R  A  X  J  S
R  N  C  S  I  P  I  L  X  Z  R  U  E  S  R
E  C  H  Y  Y  C  T  I  G  T  C  A  E  C  R
B  E  I  H  W  K  A  U  W  I  Q  P  X  L  H
U  Y  T  P  A  K  R  S  R  D  P  O  C  T  P
T  Z  I  M  A  S  I  H  I  C  C  E  C  E  T
I  X  S  E  R  N  P  E  R  T  U  S  S  I  S
U  C  Y  A  N  O  S  I  S  P  A  X  I  G  W
O  D  S  L  O  Y  A  O  X  S  H  J  U  Y  P
```

▶ CASE STUDIES

1. A patient is transported to the imaging department by wheelchair for a "two view erect chest series." The patient is unable to stand, however, as she previously had both legs amputated.

   ▶ Discuss how you would take the required two projections of the chest in an upright position.

   ....

   ....

   ....

   ....

   ....

   ....

   ....

   ....

   ....

   ....

2. A patient is transported to the imaging department by stretcher for a chest radiograph. He has a Swan-Ganz catheter inserted in the femoral vein and is unable to bend his leg to sit in an upright position. The diagnosis is "CHF with pleural effusion on the right side."

   ▶ Discuss how you would take the required two projections of the chest without bending the patient's leg.

   ▶ Describe how the patient might be positioned to best visualize the pleural effusion on the radiograph.

   ▶ Explain how the pleural effusion would look on the completed radiographs.

   ....

   ....

   ....

   ....

   ....

   ....

   ....

   ....

   ....

   ....

   ....

▶ POSITIONING WORKSHEETS

COLOR THE KIDNEYS, LARGE INTESTINE, AND BONY ANATOMY EACH A DIFFERENT COLOR AND LABEL THE FOLLOWING ANATOMICAL PARTS ON THE DRAWINGS FOR THIS SECTION. LABEL ALL PARTS THAT CAN BE SEEN ON EACH POSITION OR PROJECTION.

ABDOMEN: AP [KUB], AP Upright, and Left Lateral Decubitus			
▶ KIDNEYS	▶ BONY ANATOMY	Pelvis (including iliac crest)	▶ DIAPHRAGM
▶ LARGE INTESTINE	Ribs		▶ PSOAS MAJOR MUSCLES
	Vertebral column	▶ FUNDUS OF STOMACH	

COMPLETE THE APPROPRIATE INFORMATION SHEET FOR EACH DRAWING.

3

ABDOMEN

▶ AP ABDOMEN

CENTERING LANDMARK AND CR ORIENTATION

PATIENT POSITIONING

MAIN STRUCTURES VISUALIZED

NOTES

AP ABDOMEN

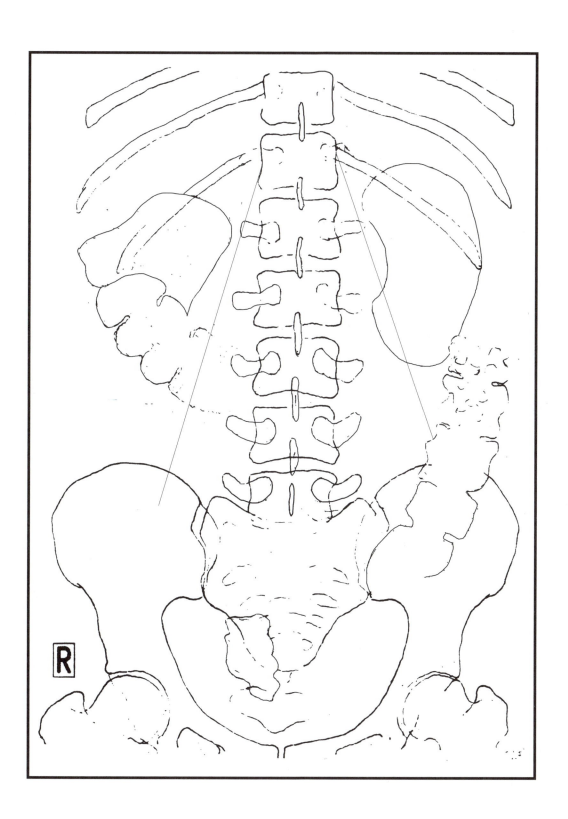

► UPRIGHT AP ABDOMEN

CENTERING LANDMARK AND CR ORIENTATION

....
....
....
....
....
....

PATIENT POSITIONING

....
....
....
....
....
....

MAIN STRUCTURES VISUALIZED

....
....
....
....
....

NOTES

....
....
....
....
....
....

UPRIGHT AP ABDOMEN

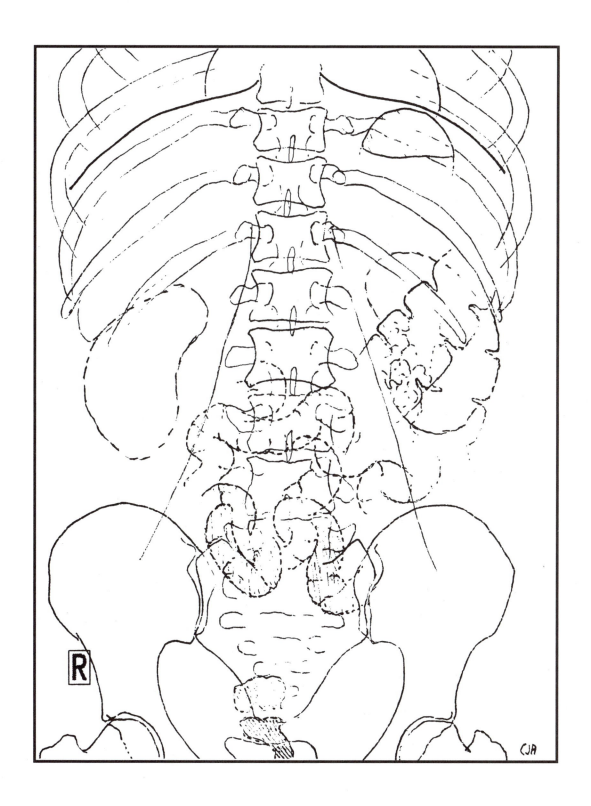

► LEFT LATERAL DECUBITUS ABDOMEN

CENTERING
LANDMARK AND CR
ORIENTATION

PATIENT
POSITIONING

MAIN STRUCTURES
VISUALIZED

NOTES

LEFT LATERAL DECUBITUS ABDOMEN

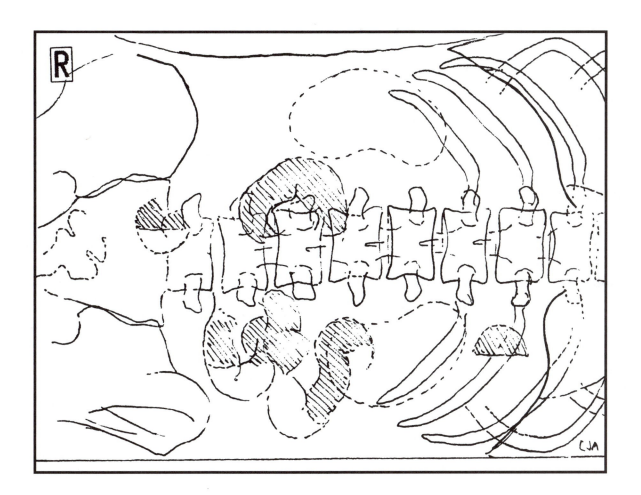

► STUDY QUESTIONS

1. The muscular _____ separates the abdominopelvic cavity from the thoracic cavity.

2. The double-walled membrane lining the abdominopelvic cavity is the _____ .

3. Double-layered tissues that stretch from the abdominal walls to the abdominal organs to support them and hold them in place are known as the _____ and _____ .

4. Identify the nine regions of the abdominopelvic cavity.

_____ _____ _____

_____ _____ _____

_____ _____ _____

5. In which of the nine regions is the spleen located? _____
_____

6. Identify the four quadrants of the abdomen.

_____   _____

_____   _____

7. In which quadrant is the appendix located? _____

8. In which quadrant is the gallbladder located? _____

9. How does a person's body habitus affect his/her abdominopelvic cavity? _____
_____
_____

10. There are _____ thoracic vertebrae, although only the lower one or two are actually in the abdominopelvic cavity.

11. Describe the location of the vertebral column in the abdominopelvic cavity. _____
_____

12. Which division of the vertebral column is described as having bodies that are large and boxlike? _____
_____

13. The _____ is comprised of five fused vertebrae and is shaped like a shovel.

14. The _____ is also known as the tailbone.

15. What structures on the lumbar vertebrae can be palpated on the patient's back? _____

16. Where are the intervertebral joints located? _____
_____

17. The _____ or wing is the upper flared portion of the ilium.

18. Relative to the vertebral column, the iliac crest corresponds to the level of the _____
_____ .

19. A palpable bony landmark located at the anterior edge of the iliac crest is the _____
_____ .

20. The right and left pubic bones meet medially to form the
_____ .

21. What is the name of the rounded process on the posteroinferior aspect of each ischium? _____
_____

22. The _____ foramen is the large opening found between the ischium and pubic bone.

23. Why is the symphysis pubis a useful landmark for localization of the urinary bladder? _____
_____

24. The _____ is a large palpable prominence located on the lateral margin of the proximal femur at the junction of the femoral neck and shaft.

25. What is a hemidiaphragm? _____
_____

26. The right and left _____ muscles help form the posterior wall of the abdominopelvic cavity.

27. What is the alimentary canal? _____
_____

28. Describe the location of the psoas major muscles relative to the vertebral column. _____
_____

29. The alimentary canal begins at the _____ and terminates at the _____ .

30. The esophagus passes from the thoracic cavity into the abdomen approximately at the level of _____ _____

31. The abdominal esophagus is also known as the _____ _____ and is approximately _____ _____ in length.

32. Using the nine-region method of localization, describe the location of the stomach. _____

33. Describe the characteristic shape of the stomach in a sthenic person. _____

34. _____ are folds in the mucosal lining of the stomach.

35. The _____ is the opening between the stomach and the small intestine.

36. The three main portions of the stomach are the _____ _____ , _____ , and _____ .

37. You are viewing a PA projection of the chest and notice the presence of a gas bubble under the left hemidiaphragm. In which part of the alimentary canal is this gas located? _____

38. List the three divisions of the small intestine in the correct order. _____ , _____ , and _____

39. The small intestine averages _____ in length.

40. The _____ is the 10-in. C-shaped portion of the small intestine.

41. What is the longest portion of the small intestine? _____ _____

42. In which quadrant(s) of the abdomen is the jejunum primarily located? _____ _____

43. In which quadrant(s) is the ileocecal valve generally located? _____

44. How does the placement of the large intestine within the abdomen differ from that of the small intestine? _____ _____

45. The _____ is the rounded saclike portion at the beginning of the large intestine.

46. The bend between the ascending and transverse sections of the colon is known as the _____ _____ .

47. The S-shaped segment of the colon is known as the _____ .

48. The ascending colon is located on the _____ (right/left) side of the abdominopelvic cavity.

49. Describe the appearance and location of the haustra. _____

50. The vermiform appendix is attached to the _____ _____ of the large intestine.

51. You are viewing an AP supine projection of the abdomen that demonstrates the presence of much gas. How can you determine if the gas is in the small or large intestine? ___ _____

52. What is the function of the urinary system? _____ _____

53. Why are the kidneys described as "retroperitoneal" structures? _____ _____

54. What anatomic characteristic allows the kidneys to be visible on a radiograph of the abdomen without the use of a contrast medium? _____ _____

55. Which kidney is positioned slightly lower than the other kidney? Explain your answer. _____ _____

56. Urine drains from the kidneys to the urinary bladder via the_____ .

57. Describe the location of the urinary bladder. _____
_____

58. Name the structures of the endocrine system that are located superiorly and medially to each kidney. _____
_____

59. The liver is located under the _____ (right/left) hemidiaphragm.

60. The _____ functions to store, concentrate, and release bile.

61. The _____ duct transports bile to the duodenum of the small intestine.

62. What structure is responsible for the production of bile?
_____

63. The _____ duct transports bile into and out of the gallbladder.

64. Why is it difficult and often impossible to apply lead shielding for abdominal radiography of a female patient?
_____
_____

65. Describe the location of the uterus relative to the urinary bladder and rectum. _____
_____

66. As the female gonads, the _____ produce eggs (ova) and secrete sexual hormones.

67. A surgical procedure in which the uterine tubes are cut or tied off to prevent pregnancy is a/an _____
_____ .

68. Surgical removal of the uterus is known as a/an _____
_____ .

69. Ova are transported to the uterus by the _____
_____ _____ .

70. The male reproductive gonads are the two _____
_____ _____ .

71. Is it possible to shield the male reproductive organs when taking an AP projection of the abdomen? Explain your answer. _____
_____

72. The _____ is located just inferior to the symphysis pubis and encircles the proximal portion of the male urethra.

73. The _____ secretes hormones that regulate the concentration of sugar in the blood, and also produces enzymes that aid in digestion of food.

74. Describe the location of the spleen relative to the stomach and kidneys. _____
_____

75. The largest artery in the abdomen is the _____
_____ .

76. The largest vein in the abdomen is the _____
_____ .

77. Which organ in the abdominopelvic cavity plays an important role in the formation and storage of blood cells?
_____

78. A condition in which the organs of the abdominopelvic cavity are reversed, such as a left-sided liver, is known as
_____ .

79. A/an _____ is a surgical procedure that involves the introduction of an endoscope through an incision in the abdominal wall.

80. Why is it recommended that a patient remove his/her underpants prior to radiography of the abdomen? _____
_____

81. When taking an upright or decubitus projection of the abdomen, why should a patient be in the position for a minimum of 10 minutes prior to the exposure? _____
_____

82. What is a "KUB"? _____

83. What is the purpose of placing a pillow or sponge under the patient's knees when taking an AP supine projection of the abdomen? _____
_____

84. What is the centering point for a recumbent AP projection of the abdomen? _____
_____

85. When positioning for a PA projection of the abdomen, how can you assure that the urinary bladder will be included on the radiograph? _____ _____

86. What projections can the radiographer take to demonstrate the presence of free air in the abdominopelvic cavity? _____ _____

87. You have a requisition to perform an acute abdominal series and PA upright chest on a patient who was transported to the radiology department by wheelchair. Which projection will you take first? Explain your answer. _____ _____

88. What is an *acute abdominal series?* _____ _____ _____

89. What is the centering point for an upright projection of the abdomen? _____ _____

90. You are viewing a left lateral decubitus projection of the abdomen. How can you determine if rotation is present on the radiograph? _____ _____

91. A dorsal decubitus projection of the abdomen taken on an elderly patient demonstrated a calcified abdominal aorta. Describe the location of the aorta on the radiograph. _____ _____

92. What range of kVp is recommended for radiography of the abdomen? _____

93. A/an _____ is the radiographic examination of the female reproductive system (uterus and uterine tubes) after the injection of _____ contrast medium.

94. Why is a left lateral decubitus projection of the abdomen taken to demonstrate the presence of free air rather than a right lateral decubitus projection? _____ _____

INDICATE TRUE OR FALSE FOR QUESTIONS 95–99.

_____ 95. A supine radiograph of the abdomen may be taken to check for residual contrast medium from an earlier examination of the GI tract.

_____ 96. Radiographs of the abdomen should be taken on inhalation so that the diaphragm can be included on the films.

_____ 97. On a properly exposed radiograph of the abdomen, the renal shadows, inferior margin of the liver, psoas major muscles, and transverse processes of the lumbar vertebrae should be visible.

_____ 98. A gunshot wound to the abdomen may result in the presence of free air under the left hemidiaphragm on an upright projection.

_____ 99. The use of a grid is required for radiography of the abdomen.

100. Complete the following table:

Projection	CR Angle/Angle of Part	Centering Point	Film Size	Structures Seen
PA recumbent abdomen				
AP upright abdomen				
Left lateral decubitus abdomen				

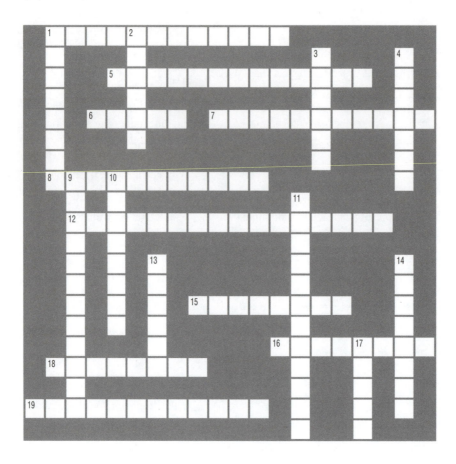

ACROSS

1. Inability to control urination
5. Surgical procedure in which the uterine tubes are cut or tied off to prevent pregnancy
6. Obstruction of the intestines, specifically the small intestine
7. Wavelike movement
8. Endoscopic examination of the abdomen
12. Condition in which air or gas is present in the peritoneal cavity
15. Yellow discoloration of the skin, usually due to a disorder of the gallbladder or liver
16. Formation of a stone
18. Constriction or a body opening or passage
19. Surgical removal of the uterus

DOWN

1. Type of hernia in which the intestines protrude through the abdominal wall
2. Sick feeling that may result in vomiting
3. Type of hernia in which a portion of the stomach protrudes up through the esophageal opening of the diaphragm
4. Abnormal accumulation of fluid in the peritoneal cavity
9. Inflammation of the appendix
10. A dorsal decubitus projection may be taken to demonstrate this condition in which a weakened area in the wall of the abdominal aorta balloons outward
11. Difficulty in eliminating fecal material
13. Vomiting
14. Twisting of the intestine that results in obstruction
17. Hollow or craterlike lesion on the surface of an organ or tissue

► CASE STUDIES

1. The history on 3-year-old Desmond indicated that "Grandma gave him a quarter for being a good boy; however, Desmond swallowed the quarter. He does not appear to have any breathing difficulties." The child's pediatrician ordered a KUB on the child, but requested that the area from the mouth to anus be included on the film.

   ► Where will you center to include the anatomy of interest?

   ► The AP projection reveals a foreign body in the region of the neck. How will you determine if it is in the airway or the esophagus?

2. The patient's radiographic request asks for an upright and supine abdomen series to visualize a very small amount of free air in the peritoneum. The patient arrives on a stretcher; she is vomiting and in obvious pain.

   ► Describe how you would take the radiographs that were ordered.

   ► Discuss the patient's physical condition and the possible concerns you may have regarding her condition.

   ► If she is unable to sit upright, what other projection(s) could you take to demonstrate the pathology?

► STUDY QUESTIONS

1. Define *osteology*. _____

2. There are approximately _____ bones in the human skeleton.

3. List the five important functions of the skeletal system:

   A. _____

   B. _____

   C. _____

   D. _____

   E. _____

4. The two basic types of osseous tissue are _____ and _____ bone.

5. The skeleton comprises approximately _____ % of the body's mass.

6. Which type of osseous tissue has a spongelike appearance? _____
   _____

7. Where are the blood vessels, lymphatic vessels, and nerves found in the compact bone? _____

8. The sponge network in cancellous bone forms fine bony spikes called _____ .

9. The outer covering of a bone is known as _____ .

10. The _____ or shaft is the cylindrical central portion of a long bone.

11. The _____ cavity extends the length of the shaft of a long bone and is filled with _____ .

12. What is *cortical bone?* _____
    _____

13. Where is the endosteum located on a long bone? _____
    _____

14. What type of bones form the wrist? _____

15. Blood vessels are transported to the medullary cavity of a long bone by way of a _____ located on the shaft.

16. What type of bone is embedded in a tendon and develops near joints in areas of sress? _____

17. Where are wormian bones located? _____
_____

18. Name the two divisions of the skeleton: _____
_____

19. The _____ is an example of a flat bone.

20. Osteogenesis or _____ is the process of bone formation.

21. What is the metaphysis of a long bone? _____
_____
_____

22. A rapid form of bone growth, which is usually seen in flat bones, is called _____
_____ .

23. As a person grows taller, what parts of the bones of the femur, tibia, and fibula are growing? _____
_____

24. You are viewing radiographs of the knee, which another radiographer has just processed. How can you determine from the anatomy on the radiograph that the patient was a young child? _____
_____
_____

25. The secondary centers of ossification in endochondral ossification are known as _____ .

26. How is the body able to repair a fractured bone? _____
_____
_____

27. Bone-destroying cells known as _____ are responsible for breaking down old bone tissue in the process of bone resorption.

28. Mature bone cells are called _____ .

29. Radiographs are often taken of fractures of the femur to document progress of the healing process. Describe the radiographic appearance of callus. _____
_____

30. Match the following surface markings of bone with the correct definition.

A. _____ slender pointed process
B. _____ narrow slit or cleftlike opening
C. _____ shallow depression or hollow area on a bone for articulation
D. _____ prominent ridge or border
E. _____ large, rounded (roughened) process
F. _____ rounded, knucklelike process
G. _____ blunt, large projection only found on the femur
H. _____ rounded, ball-like structure above a constricted neck
I. _____ round opening for passage of blood vessels and nerves
J. _____ a hollow cavity or recess in a bone

1. condyle
2. crest
3. epicondyle
4. facet
5. fissure
6. foramen
7. fossa
8. groove
9. head
10. sinus
11. spine
12. trochanter
13. tubercle
14. tuberosity

31. A condition in which the bone becomes infected as the result of a staph infection is known as _____
_____ .

32. A/an _____ is defined as any break in the cortex of a bone.

33. Postmenopausal women are particularly susceptible to _____ , a condition in which a large amount of bone mass is lost.

34. The presence of a fracture is often obvious prior to radiography of the part. List seven physical signs that may indicate the presence of a fracture. _____
_____
_____
_____
_____
_____
_____

INDICATE THE CORRECT NAME FOR THE VARIOUS TYPES OF FRACTURES DESCRIBED IN QUESTIONS 35–39.

35. _____ fractures are chip fractures often seen in the fingers from forcible pulling or twisting, which results in tearing of the muscle or ligament attachments.

36. In a/an _____ fracture, the fractured bone protrudes through the skin.

37. A bulging fracture often seen in children is called a/an _____ fracture.

38. A/an _____ fracture occurs as the result of an injury in which the bone is twisted, such as a skiing accident.

39. A/an _____ fracture results in the bone being broken into many small fragments.

40. Define *articulation.* _____
_____

41. The three classifications of joints according to function (movement) are: _____ ,
_____ , _____

42. The bones of the skull form irregular-shaped joints called _____ .

43. A type of slightly movable joint in which the bones are separated by a pad of cartilage is known as a/an _____
_____ .

44. The joints formed by the articulation of the teeth with the bony sockets of the maxillae and mandible are called _____ and are classified according to function (movement) as _____ .

45. What is a *syndesmosis?* _____
_____
_____

46. What type of joint is found between the epiphysis and diaphysis of a long bone in a child? How does this joint change as the child matures? _____
_____
_____
_____

47. Structurally, what differentiates a diarthrodial joint from a synarthrodial joint? _____
_____
_____

48. Identify the structural and functional classifications of the hip joint. _____
_____

49. What is the function of synovial fluid? Where is it found?
_____
_____
_____

50. Articular fibrocartilaginous disks found in the knee joint to cushion and absorb shock are called _____ .

51. List the six types of movement permitted by diarthrodial joints.
_____
_____
_____
_____
_____
_____

52. Which type of diarthrodial joint permits flexion, extension, abduction, adduction, and circumduction? Give an example. _____

53. The articulation between the first and second cervical vertebrae is an example of a/an _____ joint.

54. The root *my/o-* means _____ .

55. Name the three types of muscles found in the body.
_____ , _____ ,
_____

56. What are the four primary functions of the muscular system? _____

_____

_____

_____

57. A/an _____ is a band of fibrous connective tissue that extends across a joint to bind the articulating bones together.

58. Why are skeletal muscles described as "voluntary" muscles? _____

_____

59. _____ muscles are the smooth muscles found in the walls of some organs, such as the stomach.

60. A ringlike muscle that is usually found at an orifice such as the mouth is known as a/an _____ .

61. How do the terms *origin* and *insertion* apply to a muscle?

_____

_____

_____

62. A/an _____ is a minor injury to muscle tissue that usually results from overstretching.

63. What projections should be included in a radiographic examination of any long bone? _____

_____

64. If a patient comes into the emergency department with a bruise on her shin, what information would you record for a patient history prior to radiography of the leg? _____

_____

_____

_____

65. Why is an oblique projection usually included in radiographic examinations of the joints? _____

_____

66. Pathologic conditions of the skeleton that are destructive in nature may require a/an _____ (increase / decrease) in kVp or mAs.

FOR QUESTIONS 67–71, INDICATE WHICH OF THE FOLLOWING PATHOLOGIC CONDITIONS ARE ADDITIVE OR DESTRUCTIVE IN NATURE. A = ADDITIVE D = DESTRUCTIVE

67. _____ atrophy

68. _____ callus

69. _____ Paget's disease

70. _____ gout

71. _____ osteoporosis

72. Why would the use of a small focal spot be recommended for radiography of the wrist? _____

_____

73. When are "post-reduction" radiographs taken? _____

_____

_____

74. You have a requisition to take a post-reduction wrist exam on a patient whose wrist is in a fiberglass cast. How will you modify a non-cast technique to produce an acceptable radiograph? _____

_____

75. The radiography department where you work uses slow speed "detail" cassettes for radiography of the extremities. Why is the use of these cassettes not recommended for the post-reduction exam in the previous question?

_____

_____

76. Why is the use of lower kVp often desirable for skeletal radiography of the elderly patient? _____

_____

_____

77. A patient who is undergoing renal dialysis has been sent to the radiography department for a skeletal survey. What is the purpose of such an exam? _____

_____

_____

78. _____ is a radiographic examination of the soft-tissue structures of a joint after the injection of contrast medium.

79. What is a Bone Age Study? _____
_____
_____

► WORD SEARCH

USING THE FOLLOWING CLUES, FIND TERMI-
NOLOGY RELATED TO THE MUSCULOSKELE-
TAL SYSTEM IN THE WORD SEARCH PUZZLE.

1. Fusion or fixation of joint usually resulting from inflam-matory disease or injury

2. Pain in a joint

3. Radiograph of a joint taken after the injection of contrast medium

4. Any break in the cortex of a bone

5. Process of blood cell formation; takes place in red bone marrow

6. Each vertebra is classified as this type of bone

7. The humerus is an example of this type of bone

8. Dislocation, specifically of a bone from a joint

9. The moving force behind the skeletal framework of the body

10. The study of muscles

11. Branch of medicine that deals with the function, correc-tion, and prevention of abnormalities of the muscu-loskeletal system

12. Abnormal softening of bone due to demineralization of bony tissue

13. Minor injury to muscle tissue due to overstretching

14. Type of joint found in the cranium

15. Bony network found in cancellous bone

```
S  I  D  L  L  G  E  R  U  T  U  S  M  G  J
I  G  I  S  Y  E  I  R  G  D  J  R  N  X  I
S  O  F  C  Y  R  A  L  U  G  E  R  R  I  J
E  D  G  I  H  G  J  L  M  T  N  D  N  C  A
I  N  H  D  J  U  O  Q  U  O  C  G  Q  R  I
O  S  T  E  O  M  A  L  A  C  I  A  T  Z  V
P  F  F  P  V  K  P  Q  O  L  E  H  R  L  I
O  L  L  O  N  G  S  K  U  Y  R  B  Q  F  M
T  S  S  H  G  R  V  X  S  O  M  G  A  U  K
A  A  R  T  H  R  A  L  G  I  A  T  S  R  L
M  F  T  R  R  T  Y  R  J  P  Z  C  D  K  T
E  C  F  O  I  A  A  N  K  Y  L  O  S  I  S
H  E  Q  O  B  M  I  B  M  E  N  B  E  Q  K
F  T  N  A  J  S  Z  N  S  F  D  M  D  X  M
```

▶ POSITIONING WORKSHEETS

COLOR EACH BONE OR TYPE OF BONE (IE, PHALANGES) ONE COLOR AND LABEL THE FOLLOWING ANATOMICAL PARTS ON THE DRAWINGS FOR THIS SECTION. LABEL ALL PARTS THAT CAN BE SEEN ON EACH POSITION OR PROJECTION.

HAND: PA, Oblique, Lateral

- ▶ PHALANGES
  Distal phalanx
  Middle phalanx
  Proximal phalanx

- ▶ METACARPALS
  Number 1 through 5
  Head
  Body
  Base

- ▶ CARPALS
  Color one color and label
    collectively
- ▶ RADIUS
- ▶ ULNA

- ▶ ARTICULATIONS
  Distal interphalangeal
  Proximal interphalangeal
  Metacarpophalangeal
  Carpometacarpal

WRIST: PA, PA Oblique, AP Oblique, Lateral, Ulnar Flexion

- ▶ METACARPALS
- ▶ CARPALS
  Color each carpal a
    different color
  Scaphoid (navicular)
  Lunate (semilunar)

  Triquetrum (triangular)
  Pisiform
  Trapezium (greater
    multangular)
  Trapezoid (lesser
    multangular)

  Capitate (os magnum)
  Hamate (unciform)
- ▶ RADIUS
- ▶ ULNA

- ▶ ARTICULATIONS
  Intercarpal
  Radiocarpal
  Distal radioulnar

FOREARM: AP, Lateral

- ▶ RADIUS
  Styloid process
  Shaft
  Head

  Neck
  Radial tuberosity
- ▶ ULNA
  Styloid process
  Head

  Shaft
  Olecranon process
  Trochlear (semilunar)
    notch
  Coronoid process

- ▶ HUMERUS
- ▶ ARTICULATIONS
  Distal radioulnar
  Proximal radioulnar

ELBOW: AP, Lateral, Medial Oblique, Lateral Oblique

- ▶ RADIUS
  Radial head
  Neck
  Radial tuberosity
- ▶ ULNA
  Olecranon process

  Trochlear (semilunar)
    notch
  Coronoid process
- ▶ ARTICULATIONS
  Proximal radioulnar
  Humeroulnar

  Humeroradial
- ▶ HUMERUS
  Capitulum
  Trochlea
  Olecranon fossa
  Coronoid fossa

  Medial epicondyle
  Lateral epicondyle
  Medial condyle
  Lateral condyle

HUMERUS: AP, Lateral, Transthoracic

- ▶ HUMERUS
  Capitulum
  Trochlea
  Olecranon fossa
  Coronoid fossa

  Medial and lateral
    epicondyles
  Medial and lateral
    condyles

  Shaft
  Head
  Greater tubercle
  Lesser tubercle
  Surgical neck

  Anatomic neck
- ▶ SCAPULA
  Acromion process
  Glenoid cavity

COMPLETE THE APPROPRIATE INFORMATION SHEET FOR EACH DRAWING.

5

UPPER LIMB (EXTREMITY)

► PA HAND

CENTERING LANDMARK AND CR ORIENTATION

PATIENT POSITIONING

MAIN STRUCTURES VISUALIZED

NOTES

PA HAND

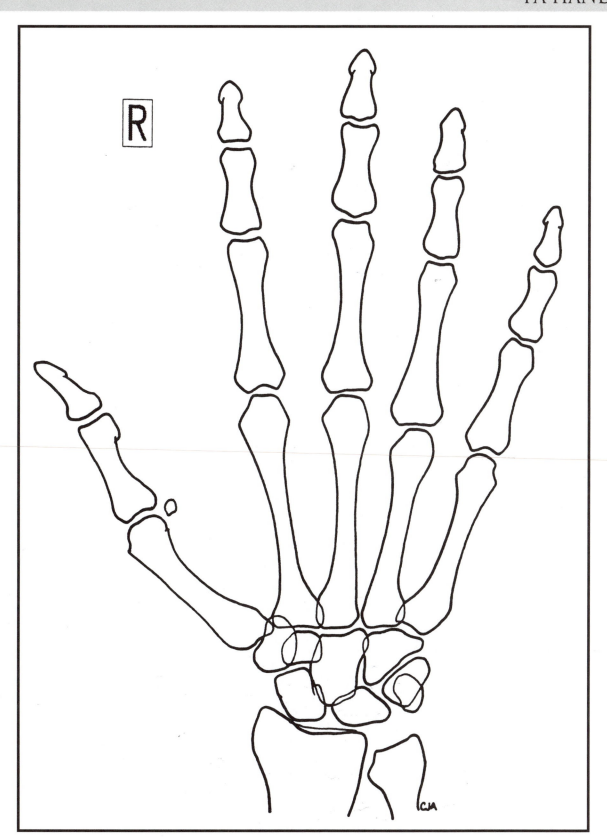

► OBLIQUE HAND

CENTERING LANDMARK AND CR ORIENTATION

PATIENT POSITIONING

MAIN STRUCTURES VISUALIZED

NOTES

OBLIQUE HAND

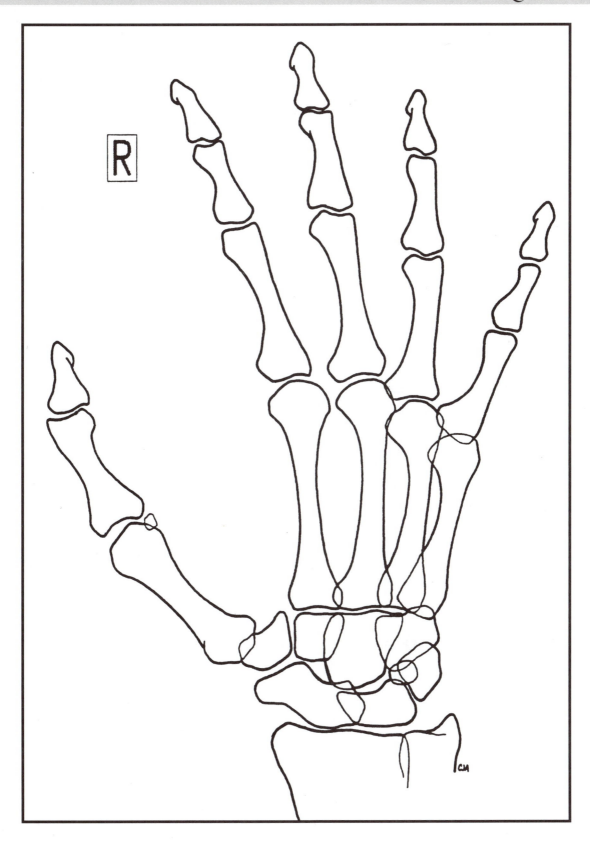

▶ LATERAL HAND

CENTERING LANDMARK AND CR ORIENTATION

PATIENT POSITIONING

MAIN STRUCTURES VISUALIZED

NOTES

LATERAL (FAN) HAND

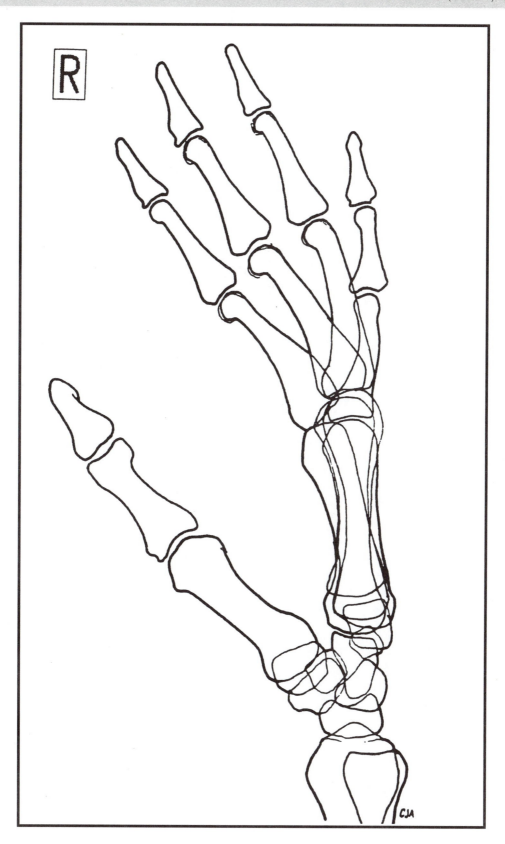

▶ PA WRIST

CENTERING LANDMARK AND CR ORIENTATION

PATIENT POSITIONING

MAIN STRUCTURES VISUALIZED

NOTES

PA WRIST

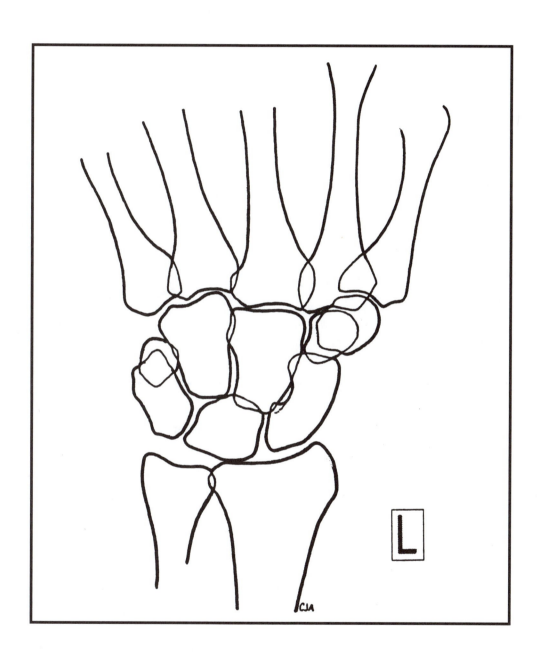

► LATERAL WRIST

CENTERING LANDMARK AND CR ORIENTATION

PATIENT POSITIONING

MAIN STRUCTURES VISUALIZED

NOTES

LATERAL WRIST

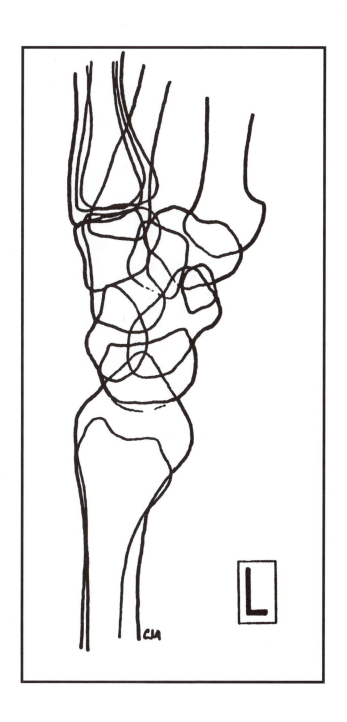

► PA OBLIQUE WRIST

CENTERING LANDMARK AND CR ORIENTATION

PATIENT POSITIONING

MAIN STRUCTURES VISUALIZED

NOTES

PA OBLIQUE WRIST

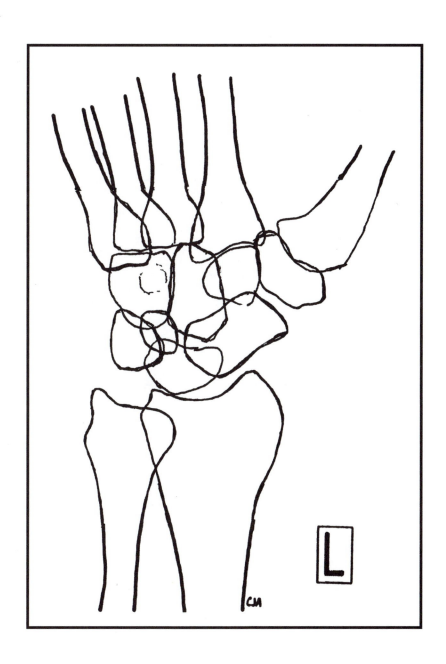

► AP OBLIQUE WRIST

CENTERING LANDMARK AND CR ORIENTATION

....
....
....
....
....
....

PATIENT POSITIONING

....
....
....
....
....
....
....

MAIN STRUCTURES VISUALIZED

....
....
....
....
....
....

NOTES

....
....
....
....
....
....
....

AP OBLIQUE WRIST

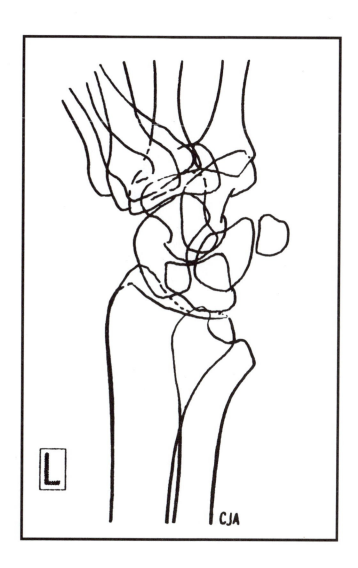

▶ ULNAR FLEXION (NAVICULAR) WRIST

CENTERING
LANDMARK AND CR
ORIENTATION

PATIENT
POSITIONING

MAIN STRUCTURES
VISUALIZED

NOTES

ULNAR FLEXION (NAVICULAR) WRIST

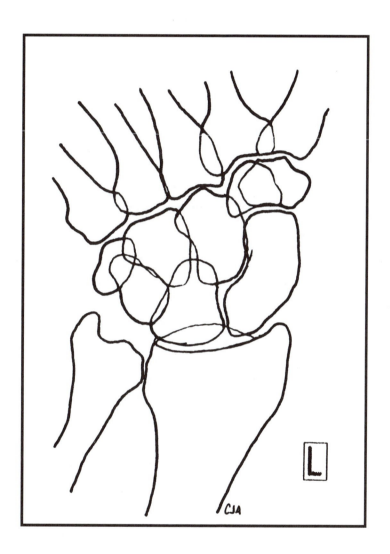

▶ LATERAL FOREARM

CENTERING
LANDMARK AND CR
ORIENTATION

....
....
....

PATIENT
POSITIONING

....
....
....

MAIN STRUCTURES
VISUALIZED

....
....
....

▶ AP FOREARM

CENTERING
LANDMARK AND CR
ORIENTATION

....
....
....

PATIENT
POSITIONING

....
....
....

MAIN STRUCTURES
VISUALIZED

....
....
....

LATERAL FOREARM   AP FOREARM

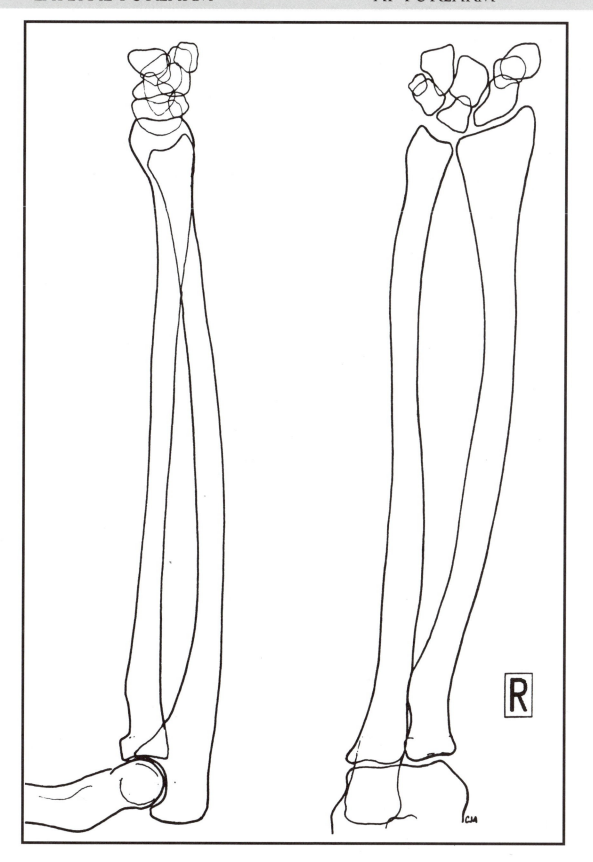

► AP ELBOW

CENTERING
LANDMARK AND CR
ORIENTATION

PATIENT
POSITIONING

MAIN STRUCTURES
VISUALIZED

NOTES

AP ELBOW

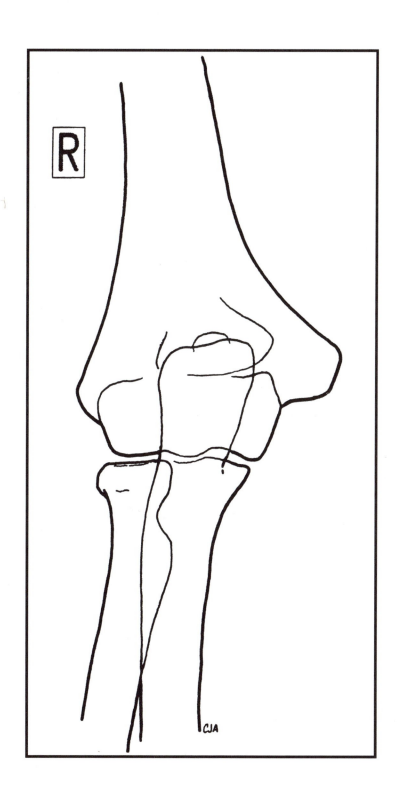

► LATERAL ELBOW

CENTERING LANDMARK AND CR ORIENTATION

PATIENT POSITIONING

MAIN STRUCTURES VISUALIZED

NOTES

LATERAL ELBOW

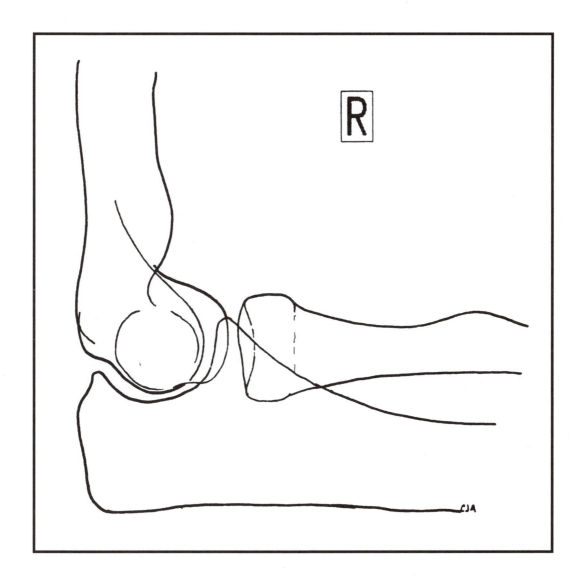

► LATERAL OBLIQUE ELBOW

CENTERING LANDMARK AND CR ORIENTATION

PATIENT POSITIONING

MAIN STRUCTURES VISUALIZED

NOTES

LATERAL (EXTERNAL) OBLIQUE ELBOW

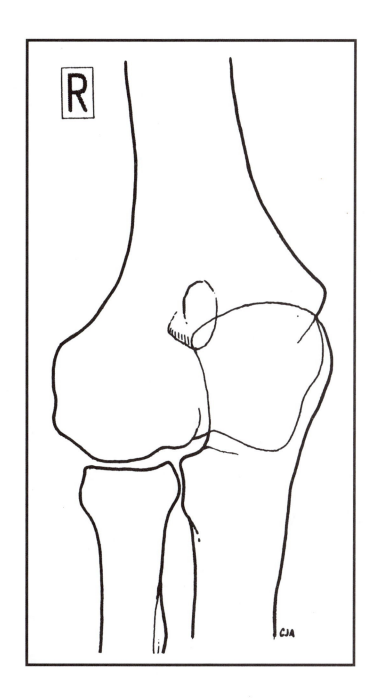

► MEDIAL OBLIQUE ELBOW

CENTERING LANDMARK AND CR ORIENTATION

PATIENT POSITIONING

MAIN STRUCTURES VISUALIZED

NOTES

MEDIAL (INTERNAL) OBLIQUE ELBOW

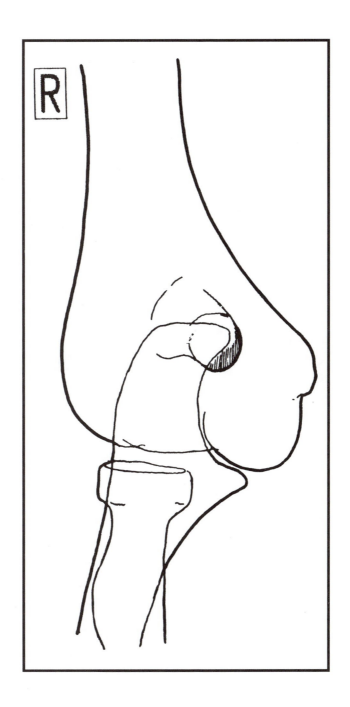

▶ AP HUMERUS

CENTERING LANDMARK AND CR ORIENTATION

....
....
....

PATIENT POSITIONING

....
....
....

MAIN STRUCTURES VISUALIZED

....
....
....

▶ LATERAL HUMERUS

CENTERING LANDMARK AND CR ORIENTATION

....
....
....

PATIENT POSITIONING

....
....
....

MAIN STRUCTURES VISUALIZED

....
....
....

AP HUMERUS   LATERAL HUMERUS

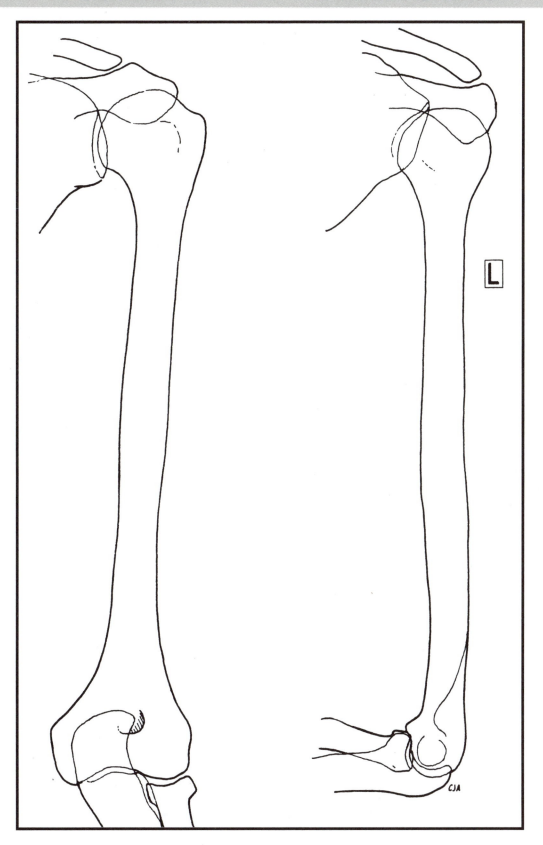

TRANSTHORACIC HUMERUS

CENTERING LANDMARK AND CR ORIENTATION

PATIENT POSITIONING

MAIN STRUCTURES VISUALIZED

NOTES

TRANSTHORACIC HUMERUS

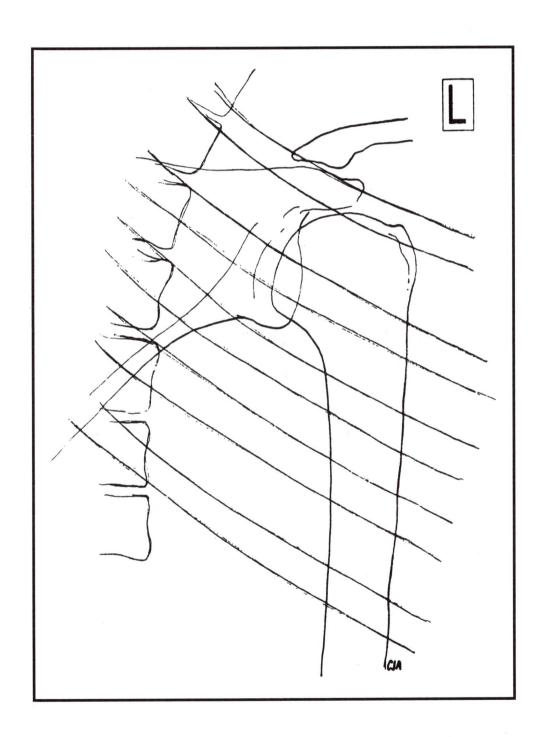

▶ STUDY QUESTIONS

1. There are _____ phalanges forming the fingers or _____ of the hand.

2. What is the tuft or ungulate process of a phalanx? _____
   _____

3. The thumb is also referred to as the _____ .

4. What type of bone are the phalanges? _____
   _____

5. The rounded _____ of the phalanx is located distally, while the more flattened _____ is found at the proximal end of the bone.

6. There are a total of _____ metacarpals in each upper limb.

7. What is the *carpus?* _____

8. On which side of the hand do you begin when naming the metacarpals? _____

9. What part of the metacarpals forms a person's knuckles when he makes a fist? _____

10. How many carpal bones form the wrist? _____

11. List the carpal bones of the distal row in order beginning on the lateral side of the wrist. _____
    _____
    _____

12. The _____ is a triangular-shaped carpal bone located on the medial side of the wrist.

13. The largest carpal bone is the _____ .
    It is also known as the _____ .

14. Which carpal bone is crescent-shaped, resembling a half moon? _____

15. The scaphoid is also called the _____ and is located on the _____ side of the wrist.

16. Why is the hamate also known as the unciform?
    _____

17. List the two names for the carpal bone that directly articulates with the thumb. _____
    and _____

18. Describe the location of the pisiform. Be specific.
    _____

19. The carpal tunnel is formed on the _____
    _____ surface of the carpus by the transverse carpal ligament.

20. Name the two bones forming the forearm. _____
    _____

21. Which of the bones of the forearm is located on the lateral side? _____

22. Name the bones forming the palm of the hand. _____
    _____

23. Name the bones involved in the formation of the elbow joint. _____

24. The base of the ulna is located at its _____ (distal / proximal) end, while the head of the ulna is located at the bone's _____ (distal / proximal) end.

25. Where is the styloid process of the ulna located? _____
    _____

26. The carpals are classified as _____ bones.

27. Is the ulnar notch located on the radius or ulna? _____
    _____

28. On which bone is the olecranon process located? _____
    _____

29. The shafts of the radius and ulna are also known as the
    _____ .

30. The olecranon process fits into the olecranon fossa of the humerus when the elbow is _____ (extended / flexed).

31. The head of the radius articulates with the ulna at the
    _____ .

32. Describe the relationship of the trochlear notch to the coronoid and olecranon processes of the ulna.

_____

_____

33. The radial head, neck, and tuberosity are located at the bone's _____ end.

34. The two processes located on the proximal end of the ulna are the _____ and _____ _____ processes.

35. Which of the processes in the above question is located on the anterior side of the ulna? _____

36. Regarding the bones of the forearm, the _____ primarily forms the wrist joint, while the _____ _____ plays a major role in the formation of the elbow joint.

37. The _____ is the rounded distal articular end of the humerus.

38. Name the three depressions found on the distal end of the humerus. _____ , _____ _____ , _____

39. The _____ is a rough prominence located on the midshaft of the humerus that serves as the site of a muscle attachement.

40. The _____ neck of the humerus is a slightly constricted area located just below the head and above the _____ neck.

41. The metacarpals articulate distally with the _____ _____ and proximally with the __ _____ .

42. The rounded process on the lateral aspect of the inferior condylar surface of the humerus is the _____ _____ , which is also known as the _____ .

43. The _____ is a pulley-shaped structure on the medial side of the inferior aspect of the humeral condyle. It articulates with the _____ _____ of the ulna.

44. The greater tubercle is situated on the _____ margin of the proximal humerus, while the lesser tubercle is located on the _____ surface of the humerus.

45. The greater and lesser tubercles are separated from each other by the _____ _____

46. Which of the epicondyles of the humerus is situated above the trochlea? _____

47. Where is the trochlear sulcus located? _____ _____

48. What structure on the humerus is known as the "funny bone" or "crazy bone"? Explain why it is called this. _____ _____

49. Structurally, all of the joints of the upper limb are _____ _____ joints and are classified according to movement as _____ joints.

50. What area of the humerus is commonly fractured? _____

51. What is the name of the joint between the bases of the middle phalanges and heads of the proximal phalanges? _____

52. Which joints of the upper limb permit the following movements: circumduction, flexion, extension, adduction, and abduction? _____ _____

53. What is the anatomical name for the shoulder joint? _____

54. The shoulder joint is classified as a _____ joint with _____ type of movement.

55. Name the joint(s) that permit(s) the supination and pronation movements of the hand. _____ _____

56. What structure on the humerus articulates with the head of the radius? _____

57. What is the correct name for the wrist joint? _____

_____

58. What type of movement do the intercarpal joints allow?

_____

59. The elbow joint is a _____ type of di-arthrodial joint, capable of flexing and extending.

60. Describe the two articulations of the humerus that form the elbow joint. _____

_____

61. Correctly name the joint formed by the articulation of the phalanges in the left thumb. _____

_____

62. Correctly name the joint formed between the proximal phalanx of the 3rd digit and the 3rd metacarpal of the left hand. _____

_____

FOR QUESTIONS 63–72, MATCH THE FOLLOW-ING JOINTS WITH THEIR TYPE OF MOVEMENT.

H = hinge   S = saddle   G = gliding
P = pivot   B = ball and socket C = condylar

63. _____ distal radioulnar joint

64. _____ intercarpal joint between the trapezium and trape-zoid

65. _____ distal interphalangeal joint of the 4th digit

66. _____ 1st metacarpophalangeal joint

67. _____ radiocarpal joint

68. _____ 1st carpometacarpal joint

69. _____ glenohumeral joint

70. _____ 5th carpometacarpal joint

71. _____ humero-ulnar joint

72. _____ 3rd metacarpophalangeal joint

73. You have a requisition for a forearm exam. The patient's arm is splinted on a board and wrapped in an elastic ban-dage. How will you commence with the procedure?

_____

_____

_____

74. Explain the use of lead masking in radiography of the upper limb (extremity). _____

_____

75. When radiographing the forearm in the lateral position, why is it important that the shoulder lie on the same plane as the wrist? _____

_____

_____

76. What are the routine projections for a forearm? _____

_____

77. What are the routine projections for a hand? _____

_____

78. Detail (slow speed) cassettes are often recommended for radiography of the wrist but not for the humerus. Ex-plain the reasoning behind this. _____

_____

79. What is the centering point for a PA projection of the 3rd digit? _____

_____

80. An average of _____ kVp is gener-ally used for radiography of the fingers.

81. When radiographing a digit, how much of the adjacent metacarpal should be included in the collimated field?

_____

82. You are viewing a hand series that you just completed. How can rotation be determined on the PA projection?

_____

_____

83. What joints are included on an oblique projection of the 2nd digit? _____

_____

84. On an oblique projection, the finger is rotated _____ ° (degrees).

85. When performing a lateral projection of the index finger (2nd digit), how can you achieve the shortest OID?

_____

_____

86. On which projection of the fingers will the posterior aspect of the phalanges appear straight and the anterior aspect appear concave? _____

_____

87. When viewing a radiograph of the hand, how can you determine if you have the proper density on the film?

_____

_____

88. Why should an AP projection of the forearm always be taken with the hand in supination? _____

_____

89. The centering point for an oblique projection of the hand is _____

_____

90. As you view an oblique projection of the hand, you notice that the 2nd–4th digits appear curved, the distal phalanges are foreshortened, and the interphalangeal joints are closed. What is the positioning error? _____

_____

91. Which projection of the hand will best demonstrate anterior or posterior dislocation of fractures? _____

_____

92. Why should a patient be instructed to cup his or her hand for a PA projection of the wrist? _____

_____

93. A pregnant woman fell, injuring her wrist. The ER physician wants a very limited series on her and asks that you take any two projections that will best demonstrate the scaphoid area of the wrist. What will you take? _____

_____

94. The wrist should be rotated approximately _____ ° (degrees) for an AP oblique projection.

95. Describe the position of the elbow on a lateral projection of the forearm. _____

_____

96. On a tangential projection of the carpal canal, the central ray should be angled _____ ° (degrees) toward the long axis of the hand to a point 1 in. distal to the base of the _____ .

97. How much of the distal humerus and proximal forearm should be included on projections of the elbow? _____

_____

98. Why are two projections necessary when the elbow cannot be extended fully for an AP projection? _____

_____

_____

99. The recommended range of kVp for projections of the elbow is _____ kVp.

100. The entire arm should be rotated approximately _____ ° (degrees) for medial and lateral oblique projections of the elbow.

101. When evaluating radiographs of the elbow, how can correct rotation of the lateral (external) oblique projection of the elbow be determined? _____

_____

102. Describe the location of the radial head on a lateral projection of the elbow. What is the purpose of angling 45° toward the shoulder on an axial lateral projection?

_____

_____

103. Describe the appearance of the distal humerus and its relationship to the forearm on a lateral projection of the forearm, elbow, or humerus. _____

_____

_____

104. The olecranon process of the ulna is demonstrated in profile on a/an _____ projection of the elbow.

105. What are the routine projections of the humerus?
_____

106. What projections of the humerus will you take in the case of a suspected fracture or the patient's inability to rotate the arm? _____

_____

107. Why is a breathing technique recommended on a transthoracic lateral projection of the humerus? _____

_____

FOR QUESTIONS 108–112, INDICATE WHICH PROJECTION OF THE UPPER LIMB WILL DEMONSTRATE THE FOLLOWING ANATOMY.

108. The heads of the 3rd, 4th, and 5th metacarpals are slightly superimposed with space between the shafts of these three bones. A small space is seen between the heads of the 2nd and 3rd metacarpals. _____

_____

109. The carpal bones are demonstrated in an arch arrangement. _____

110. The radius and ulna lie parallel to each other; both the wrist and elbow joints are included in the collimated field. _____

111. The coronoid process of the ulna is demonstrated free of superimposition; the distal humerus, proximal radius, and proximal ulna are included on the film. _____

_____

112. The lesser tubercle is seen in profile near the glenoid cavity and the greater tubercle is superimposed over the humeral head. The entire humerus is included on the film. _____

113.   Complete the following table:

Projection	CR Angle/Angle of Part	Centering Point	Film Size	Structures Seen
Lateral hand				
Transthoracic lateral humerus				
PA wrist				
Lateral forearm				

► CASE STUDIES

1. While using an industrial sewing machine to sew leather, a woman sewed through her thumb with the needle. The needle has broken off and entered through the thumbnail, protruding through both the anterior and posterior aspects of the thumb. The wound is bleeding. The patient is being transported to the imaging department on a stretcher as she is feeling light-headed and has already fainted once. Three projections of the thumb have been ordered.

   ► What three projections will you take?

   ► Describe how you will proceed with the exam.

   ► Discuss the precautions necessary to take regarding the bleeding wound and sharp needle.

   ► Discuss the precautions necessary to take regarding the patient's physical condition.

   ....

   ....

   ....

   ....

   ....

   ....

   ....

   ....

2. An 8-year-old child has come to the imaging department for a "bone-age study." The protocol at the clinical site is a radiograph of the left hand, to include the wrist. Upon examining the patient, you note that his left arm hangs limply at his side, his left hand has only a thumb and one finger, and the wrist is misshapen.

   ▶ Describe how you will proceed with this exam.

3. You have a requisition to take a post-reduction wrist series on a patient. The wrist is immobilized in a fiberglass cast. Because the casted wrist is flexed, it is not possible to rest the anterior surface of the arm flat on the cassette.

   ▶ What projections would you normally take for a post-reduction series of the wrist?

   ▶ How will you modify the positioning to complete the procedure?

   ▶ Discuss any technical changes necessary to compensate for the fiberglass cast.

   ▶ Discuss what type of cassette should be used for this exam.

4. A 6-year-old girl fell off of her bike, striking her right arm against the street curb. She complained of pain in the proximal forearm. Swelling and tenderness were noted by the radiographer upon examination and history. AP and lateral projections of the forearm revealed a fracture of the proximal radius. The orthopedic surgeon reduced the fracture and set the arm in a plaster cast with the elbow in a flexed position. Post-reduction AP and lateral projections of the forearm were requested.

   ▶ Why did the orthopedic surgeon specifically request an AP projection when it would be much easier to take a PA projection?

   ▶ Discuss the method you would use to obtain an AP projection of the forearm on this patient.

   ▶ Discuss any technical changes necessary to compensate for the plaster cast.

   ▶ Discuss what type of cassette should be used for this exam.

5. Your patient is an 18-year-old male who fell and injured his elbow while skateboarding. Due to the pain and swelling, he is unable to extend his elbow for the AP and oblique projections. The protocol for an elbow at your clinical site includes AP, medial oblique, lateral oblique, and lateral projections.

   ▶ Explain how you would obtain the AP and lateral elbow projections.

   ▶ Discuss how you would obtain the oblique projections since the patient is unable to extend his arm.

....

....

....

....

....

....

....

....

....

6. An emergency room resident is viewing the AP and lateral radiographs you have obtained on a 12-year-old boy who tripped while roller skating. The resident is concerned about a possible fracture of the radial head and asks about the feasibility of doing a tomographic study of the elbow. The patient is able to flex and extend his elbow, and you explain that you can do at least one more radiograph to show the radial head before doing the tomograms.

   ▶ Explain how you would obtain a radiograph to visualize the radial head free of superimposition.

   ▶ Discuss any alternate positions/projections you could use to obtain a radiograph visualizing the radial head.

....

....

....

....

....

....

....

....

....

....

7. Two weeks after sustaining an injury in a water-skiing accident, a patient is sent to the radiology department for follow-up radiographs of the humerus. A large foam wedge has been positioned between the patient's arm and thorax, and ace bandages are wrapped entirely around the arm and thorax to stabilize the arm.

   ▶ Describe how you would obtain the required two projections of the humerus to include the shoulder and elbow.

   ▶ What concerns might you have about the immobilization device prior to radiography?

....

....

....

....

....

....

....

....

....

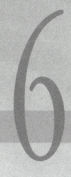

▶ POSITIONING WORKSHEETS

COLOR EACH BONE OR TYPE OF BONE ONE COLOR AND LABEL THE FOLLOWING ANATOMICAL PARTS ON THE DRAWINGS FOR THIS SECTION. LABEL ALL PARTS THAT CAN BE SEEN ON EACH POSITION OR PROJECTION.

SHOULDER: AP in Internal Rotation, AP in External Rotation, Inferosuperior Axial, PA Oblique "Y"

▶ HUMERUS
Greater tubercle
Humeral head
Anatomic neck
Surgical neck

Lesser tubercle
Intertubercular (bicipital)
  groove
▶ SCAPULA
Acromion process

Coracoid process
Glenoid cavity
▶ CLAVICLE
Acromial extremity

▶ ARTICULATIONS
Glenohumeral (scapulo
  humeral)
Acromioclavicular
Sternoclavicular

SCAPULA: AP, Lateral

▶ SCAPULA
Acromion process
Coracoid process
Scapular notch

Superior border
Medial border
Lateral border

Superior angle
Inferior angle
Neck

Glenoid cavity
▶ CLAVICLE
Acromial extremity

CLAVICLE: PA, PA Axial

CLAVICLE
Sternal extremity
Body

Acromial extremity
Conoid tubercle

▶ SCAPULA
Acromion process
Coracoid process

Superior border
Superior angle

A-C ARTICULATIONS

▶ CLAVICLE
Sternal extremity
Body

Acromial extremity
▶ SCAPULA
Acromion process

Coracoid process
▶ ARTICULATIONS
Acromioclavicular

Sternoclavicular

COMPLETE THE APPROPRIATE INFORMATION SHEET FOR EACH DRAWING.

SHOULDER GIRDLE

► AP SHOULDER IN INTERNAL ROTATION

CENTERING LANDMARK AND CR ORIENTATION

PATIENT POSITIONING

MAIN STRUCTURES VISUALIZED

NOTES

AP SHOULDER IN INTERNAL ROTATION

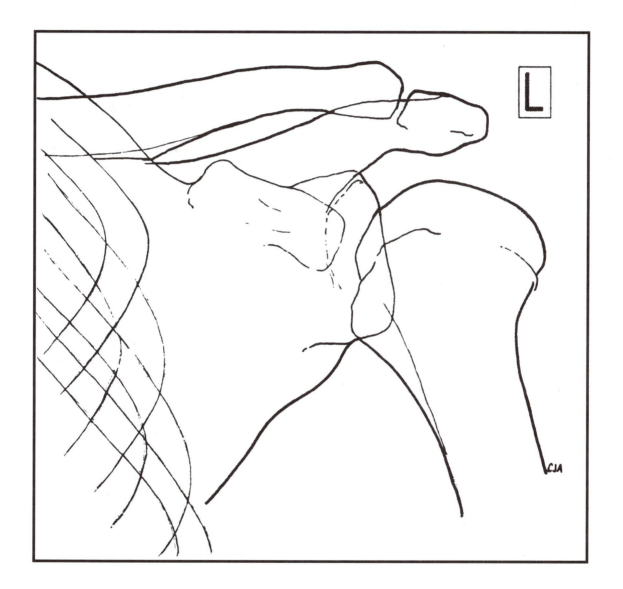

▶ AP SHOULDER IN EXTERNAL ROTATION

CENTERING
LANDMARK AND CR
ORIENTATION

PATIENT
POSITIONING

MAIN STRUCTURES
VISUALIZED

NOTES

AP SHOULDER IN EXTERNAL ROTATION

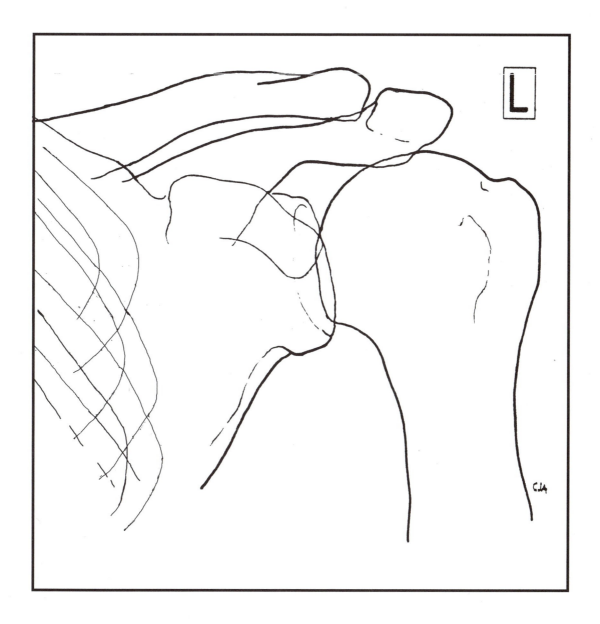

► INFEROSUPERIOR AXIAL SHOULDER

CENTERING
LANDMARK AND CR
ORIENTATION

PATIENT
POSITIONING

MAIN STRUCTURES
VISUALIZED

NOTES

INFEROSUPERIOR AXIAL SHOULDER

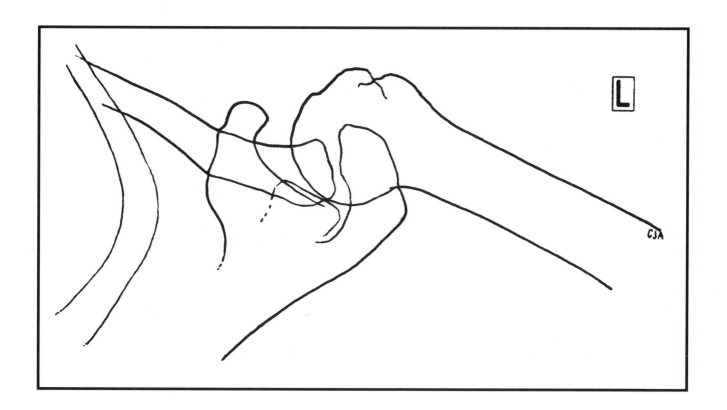

▶ PA OBLIQUE "Y" SHOULDER

CENTERING
LANDMARK AND CR
ORIENTATION

PATIENT
POSITIONING

MAIN STRUCTURES
VISUALIZED

NOTES

PA OBLIQUE "Y" SHOULDER

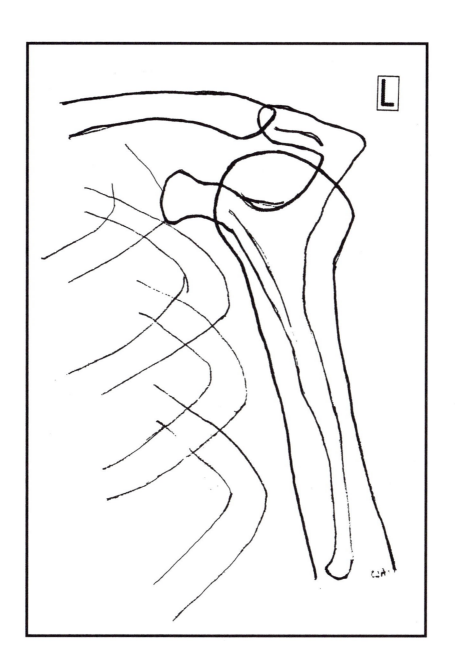

► AP SCAPULA

CENTERING LANDMARK AND CR ORIENTATION

....
....
....
....
....
....

PATIENT POSITIONING

....
....
....
....
....
....

MAIN STRUCTURES VISUALIZED

....
....
....
....
....
....

NOTES

....
....
....
....
....
....

AP SCAPULA

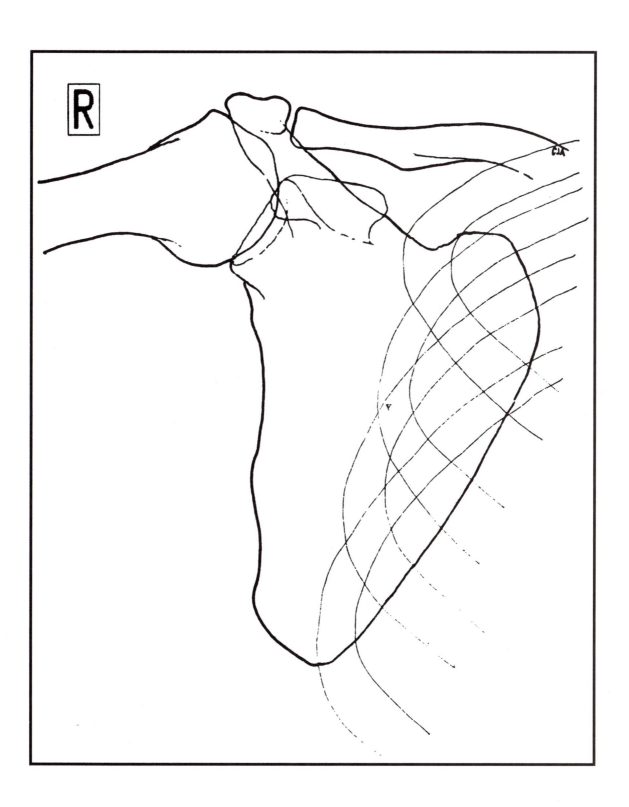

► LATERAL SCAPULA

CENTERING
LANDMARK AND CR
ORIENTATION

PATIENT
POSITIONING

MAIN STRUCTURES
VISUALIZED

NOTES

LATERAL SCAPULA

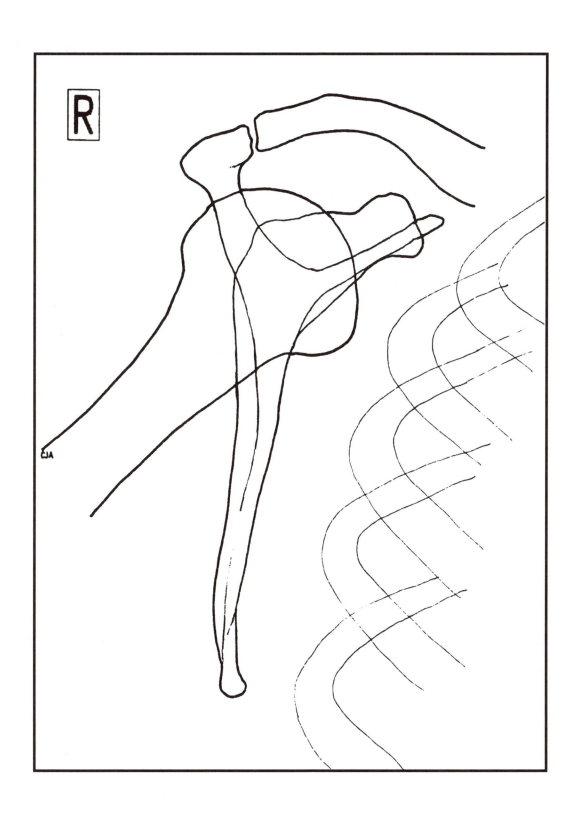

▶ PA CLAVICLE

CENTERING LANDMARK AND CR ORIENTATION

....

....

....

....

....

....

PATIENT POSITIONING

....

....

....

....

....

MAIN STRUCTURES VISUALIZED

....

....

....

....

....

NOTES

....

....

....

....

....

....

PA CLAVICLE

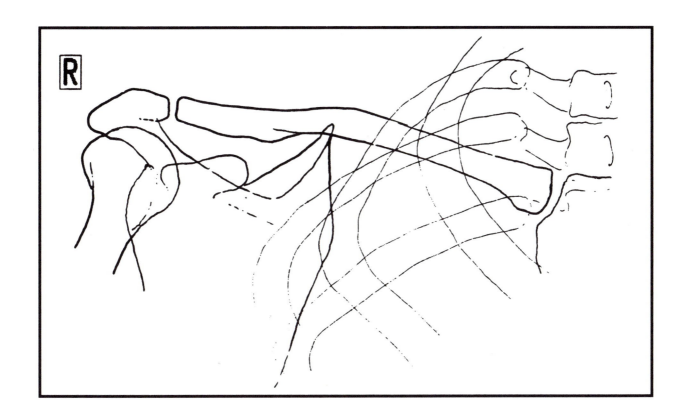

► PA AXIAL CLAVICLE

CENTERING
LANDMARK AND CR
ORIENTATION

PATIENT
POSITIONING

MAIN STRUCTURES
VISUALIZED

NOTES

PA AXIAL CLAVICLE

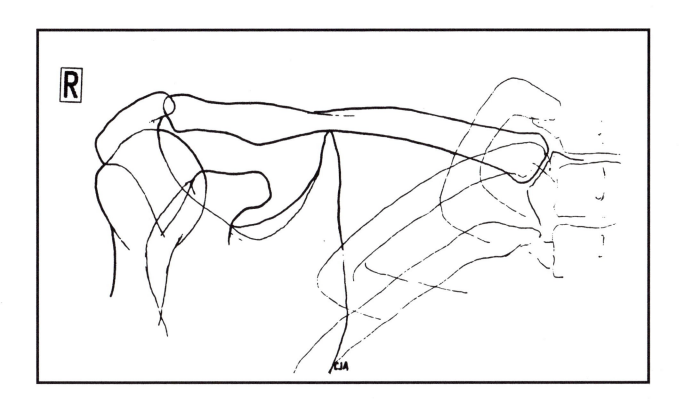

► ACROMIOCLAVICULAR ARTICULATIONS

**CENTERING
LANDMARK AND CR
ORIENTATION**

**PATIENT
POSITIONING**

**MAIN STRUCTURES
VISUALIZED**

NOTES

ACROMIOCLAVICULAR ARTICULATIONS

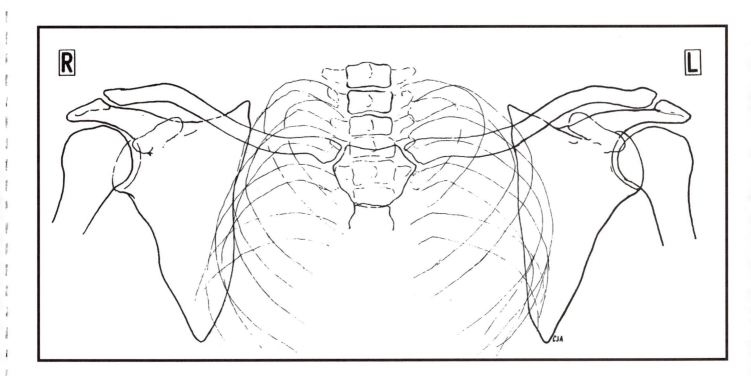

► STUDY QUESTIONS

1. Name the bones forming each shoulder girdle. _____

   _____ , _____ ,

   _____

2. What is the function of the shoulder girdle? _____

   _____

3. Which bone of the shoulder girdle does not directly artic-

   ulate with the axial skeleton? _____

4. What is the only direct articulation between the shoulder

   girdle and the axial skeleton? _____

5. In layman's terms, the clavicle is often called the _____

   _____ and the scapula is known as

   the _____ .

6. The clavicle is classified as a/an _____

   bone and the scapula is a/an _____

   bone.

7. The medial end of the clavicle is called the _____

   _____ , while the lateral end is called

   the _____ .

8. The long central portion of the clavicle is the _____

   _____ .

9. Which end of the clavicle is broader, flatter, and larger

   than the opposite end? _____

10. Describe the curvature(s) of the clavicle. _____

    _____

11. The _____ is a prominence located on

    the posteroinferior surface of the clavicle.

12. How does the clavicle act as a "brace" for the shoulder

    girdle? _____

13. The clavicles tend to be longer and more curved on _____

    _____ (females/males).

14. Describe the shape of the scapula. _____

    _____

15. Each scapula is situated laterally to the vertebral column

    between the _____ and _____

    ribs (indicate the number).

16. Name the borders of the scapula. _____

    _____

17. Which border of the scapula is adjacent to the axilla? ___

    _____

18. Where is the *ala* of the scapula located? _____

    _____

19. The anterior surface of the scapula is called the _____

    _____ or _____

    surface.

20. Which surface of the scapula is slightly concave? _____

    _____

21. The spine of the scapula is located on the bone's _____

    _____ side.

22. The extension of the spine off the lateral border of the

    scapula is called the _____ .

23. The finger- or beaklike projection that arises from the su-

    perior border of the scapula to project anteriorly is the

    _____ .

24. Where is the *scapular notch* located? _____

    _____

25. The _____ angle is located at the tip of

    the scapula.

26. The head of the scapula is located at the _____

    _____ angle.

27. The concave articular surface on the head of the scapula

    is the _____ .

28. What two structures articulate to form the "A-C" joint?

    _____

    _____

29. The superior and medial borders of the scapula meet to

    form the _____ angle.

30. Two shallow depressions located above and below the spine on the dorsal surface of the scapula are called the _____ .

31. What structure on the scapula articulates with the humerus?_____

32. What structure on the scapula projects anteriorly and can be palpated beneath the clavicle? _____

33. The _____ is a concavity on the ventral surface of the scapula in the middle of the body.

34. Name the bones and particular structures that are attached by the coracoclavicular ligament. _____

35. Explain how the scapula resembles the letter "Y". _____ _____

36. Structurally, the joints of the shoulder girdle are _____ _____ and are classified according to movement as _____ .

37. The two bones of the shoulder girdle articulate with each other and other bony structures to form a total of _____ _____ joints.

38. What is the anatomical name for the shoulder joint?_____ _____

39. The shoulder joint is classified as a _____ joint with _____ type of movement.

40. What type of movement is allowed by the sternoclavicular joints? _____

41. Name the only articulation formed between the two bones of the shoulder girdle. _____

42. Referring to the joint identified in the previous question, what type of injury commonly affects the joint after a direct blow (eg, a tackle in a football game)? _____ _____

43. The two structures forming the shoulder joint are the ____ _____ and the _____ .

44. The acromioclavicular joint has _____ type of movement.

45. Which joint of the shoulder girdle exhibits the greatest range of motion? _____

46. What are the dressing instructions for a radiographic examination of the scapula? _____ _____

47. What are the routine projections for a radiographic examination of the clavicle? _____ _____

48. A soccer player was accidentally kicked in the shoulder and has a possible separation injury of the right acromioclavicular joint. What projections are necessary to demonstrate this injury? _____ _____

49. Why shouldn't the shoulder be rotated internally or externally when there is a possible fracture of the proximal humerus? _____ _____

50. What is the purpose of abducting the arm 90° for an AP projection of the scapula? _____ _____

51. An elderly male patient was sent to the radiology department for radiographs of his shoulder. He had no history of traumatic injury, but complained of a burning pain in his shoulder. He was unable to move his arm, which was hanging at his side. What projections would you take to complete a shoulder series on him? _____ _____

52. For a weight-bearing projection of the acromioclavicular joints, a weight weighing approximately _____ pounds should hang from each of the patient's wrists.

53. The range of kVp recommended for radiography of the shoulder is fairly wide, varying from 60 to 75. When are you likely to use 60 kVp and when would you select 75 kVp for AP projections of the shoulder? _____ _____

54. Why is a 72-in. SID used for radiography of the acromio-clavicular joints? _____

_____

55. What projection(s) would be useful in identifying anterior or posterior dislocations of the shoulder? _____

_____

56. Explain why a radiographic examination of the acromio-clavicular joints should always include both the right and left joints? _____

_____

57. What are the recommended breathing instructions for radiography of the acromioclavicular joints? Explain your answer. _____

_____

58. How will you demonstrate the A-C joints bilaterally if the patient's shoulders are very broad? _____

_____

59. Examination of the A-C joints, right shoulder and clavicle have been ordered on a carpenter who fell 20 ft from a scaffold. In what order will you complete the exams? Explain your answer. _____

_____

_____

60. Describe the position of the patient's hand on an AP projection of the shoulder in external rotation. _____

_____

61. On an AP projection of the shoulder in internal rotation, the central ray is directed to the _____ .

62. Which routine projection of the shoulder will demonstrate the greater tubercle of the humerus in profile? _____

_____

63. The lesser tubercle is in profile against the glenoid cavity on a/an _____ projection.

64. What is best demonstrated (critical anatomy) on the inferosuperior axial projection of the shoulder? _____

_____

65. Describe the centering and angulation of the central ray on the inferosuperior axial projection of the shoulder.

_____

66. On the PA oblique "Y" projection of the shoulder, the midcoronal plane of the patient is rotated approximately _____ ° (degrees) to the plane of the film.

67. The ER physician suspects an anterior dislocation of the shoulder. How will this condition be demonstrated on the PA oblique "Y" projection? What structure is actually dislocated? _____

_____

68. Your patient is able to lie prone for radiographs of his clavicle. How will you determine the direction and degree of angulation of the central ray for the PA axial projection? _____

_____

69. What breathing instructions will you give a patient for an AP axial projection of the clavicle? Explain your answer.

_____

INDICATE TRUE OR FALSE FOR QUESTIONS 70–74.

_____ 70. Radiographic examinations of the scapula should be performed only in the upright position.

_____ 71. The use of a grid is recommended for the routine projections of the shoulder.

_____ 72. A sling should be removed prior to radiography of the shoulder, particularly in the case of a suspected fracture of the proximal humerus where pins or buckles could create artifacts.

_____ 73. Quiet breathing is recommended on the lateral projection of the scapula to blur the lungs and ribs.

_____ 74. When evaluating an AP projection of the scapula for positioning, the film is repeatable if the medial half of the scapula is under the rib cage.

75. Complete the following table:

Projection	CR Angle/Angle of Part	Centering Point	Film Size	Structures Seen
AP shoulder in internal rotation				
PA oblique "Y" shoulder				
AP axial clavicle				
Lateral scapula				
AP A-C joints with weights				

► CASE STUDIES

1. An elderly woman has fallen and fractured her forearm and the surgical neck of her humerus. Her forearm was casted to include the elbow in a flexed position. The arm is immobilized in a sling. She is sent as an outpatient to the radiology department for follow-up films 2 weeks later. The orthopedic surgeon is concerned about the alignment and healing of the humeral fracture and has specifically order two shoulder radiographs 90° apart.

    ► Describe the two radiographs you would obtain to demonstrate the proximal humerus.

    ► How will you make the determination whether to radiograph the patient in the recumbent or upright position?

    ► Why do you have to be concerned about rotational movement of the patient's arm?

2. A heavily sedated patient is transported to the department by stretcher. The requisition states that this patient has been diagnosed with breast cancer and has recently experienced pain in the region of her left scapula. A radiographic examination of the scapula is requested to rule out possible metastasis. The patient is unable to sit up or lie in the prone position.

    ► Explain how you would accomplish the required to projections of the scapula.

    ► What concerns might you have regarding the patient's condition?

3. Your next patient has been sent from the psychiatric unit. A radiographic examination of the right clavicle has been ordered to evaluate a large bruise and bump in the area of the right clavicle. The patient was previously diagnosed with paranoid schizophrenia and is somewhat anxious about having radiographs taken. He refuses to lie on the radiographic table and does not want to turn his back toward you.

   ▶ What projections must you take to adequately demonstrate the clavicle?

   ▶ How must you modify positioning to accommodate the patient's concerns?

   ▶ Discuss how you will proceed with this case.

4. You are listening to the radio on a quiet Saturday afternoon while working at the University Hospital. You hear that a college football player has been injured during the game, and the announcer says that the player has a "possible shoulder separation." After arriving in the emergency department, the football player is sent to radiology for examination of the A-C joints. When you see the patient, you realize that his A-C joints will not fit crosswise on a 14 × 17-in. film, even if you use 72-in. SID.

   ▶ Describe how you would radiograph both A-C joints simultaneously.

   ▶ Why is it necessary to demonstrate both A-C joints if the player injured only his right side?

► POSITIONING WORKSHEETS

COLOR EACH BONE OR TYPE OF BONE (IE, METATARSALS) ONE COLOR AND LABEL THE FOLLOWING ANATOMICAL PARTS ON THE DRAWINGS FOR THIS SECTION. LABEL ALL PARTS THAT CAN BE SEEN ON EACH POSITION OR PROJECTION.

FOOT: AP, Medial Oblique, Lateral

► PHALANGES	Body	Navicular (scaphoid)	► ARTICULATIONS
Distal phalanx	Base	Medial cuneiform	Distal interphalangeal
Middle phalanx	► TARSALS	Intermediate cuneiform	Proximal interphalangeal
Proximal phalanx	Calcaneus (os calcis)	Lateral cuneiform	Metatarsophalangeal
► METATARSALS	Talus (astragalus)	► TIBIA	Tarsometatarsal
Head	Cuboid	► FIBULA	

CALCANEUS (OS CALCIS): Axial Plantodorsal, Lateral

► CALCANEUS (OS CALCIS)	► NAVICULAR (SCAPHOID)	► TALUS (ASTRAGALUS)	► ARTICULATIONS
	► CUBOID		Talocalcaneal

ANKLE: AP, Medial Oblique, Lateral

► TIBIA	► TARSALS	Calcaneus	► ARTICULATIONS
Medial malleolus	Talus	► BASE OF 5TH	Tibiotalar
► FIBULA	Navicular	METATARSAL	Talofibular
Lateral malleolus	Cuboid		Distal tibiofibular

LOWER LEG: AP, Lateral

► TIBIA	Tibial tuberosity	Apex (styloid process)	► TALUS
Medial malleolus	Anterior border	Neck	► ARTICULATIONS
Shaft	► FIBULA	► FEMUR	Distal tibiofibular
Lateral condyle	Lateral malleolus	Medial condyle	Proximal tibiofibular
Medial condyle	Shaft	Lateral condyle	
Intercondylar eminence	Head		

KNEE: AP, Lateral, Obliques, Intercondylar Fossa, Tangential Patella

► FEMUR	► TIBIA	► PATELLA	► ARTICULATIONS
Medial condyle	Tibial plateau	Apex	Proximal tibiofibular
Lateral condyle	Intercondylar eminence	Base	Knee
Medial epicondyle	Medial condyle	► FIBULA	
Lateral epicondyle	Lateral condyle	Apex (styloid process)	
Intercondylar fossa	Tibial tuberosity	Neck	

FEMUR: AP, Lateral

► FEMUR	Lesser trochanter	Medial condyle	Apex
Head	Shaft	Lateral condyle	► TIBIA
Neck	Medial epicondyle	► PATELLA	► FIBULA
Greater trochanter	Lateral epicondyle	Base	

COMPLETE THE APPROPRIATE INFORMATION SHEET FOR EACH DRAWING.

7

LOWER LIMB (EXTREMITY)

► AP FOOT

CENTERING LANDMARK AND CR ORIENTATION

PATIENT POSITIONING

MAIN STRUCTURES VISUALIZED

NOTES

AP FOOT

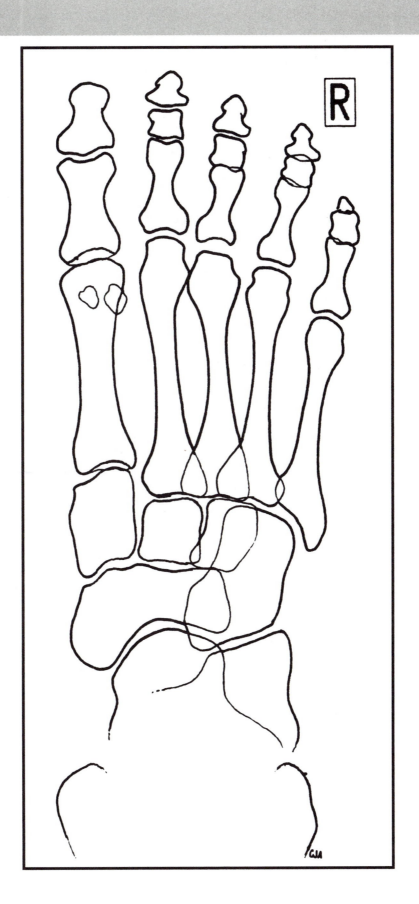

► MEDIAL OBLIQUE FOOT

CENTERING
LANDMARK AND CR
ORIENTATION

PATIENT
POSITIONING

MAIN STRUCTURES
VISUALIZED

NOTES

MEDIAL OBLIQUE FOOT

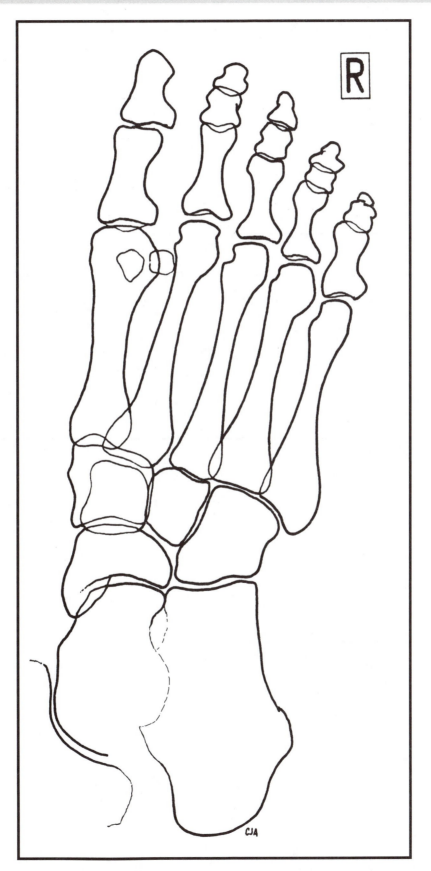

► LATERAL FOOT

CENTERING LANDMARK AND CR ORIENTATION

PATIENT POSITIONING

MAIN STRUCTURES VISUALIZED

NOTES

LATERAL FOOT

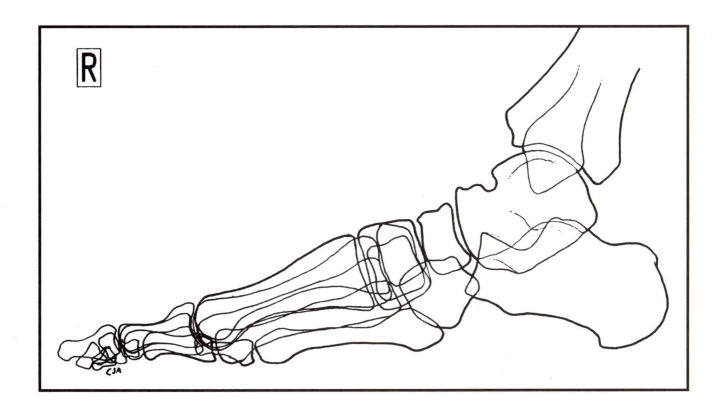

▶ AXIAL PLANTODORSAL CALCANEUS (OS CALCIS)

CENTERING LANDMARK AND CR ORIENTATION

PATIENT POSITIONING

MAIN STRUCTURES VISUALIZED

NOTES

AXIAL PLANTODORSAL CALCANEUS (OS CALCIS)

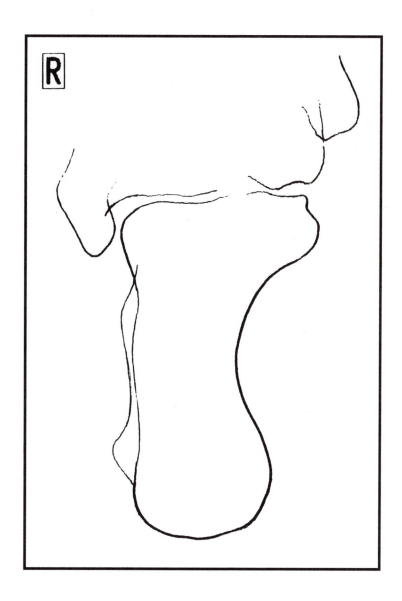

► LATERAL CALCANEUS (OS CALCIS)

CENTERING
LANDMARK AND CR
ORIENTATION

PATIENT
POSITIONING

MAIN STRUCTURES
VISUALIZED

NOTES

LATERAL CALCANEUS (OS CALCIS)

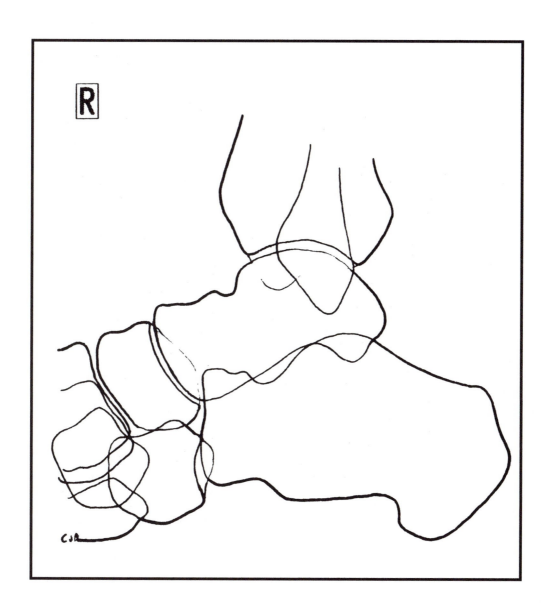

▶ AP ANKLE

CENTERING
LANDMARK AND CR
ORIENTATION

PATIENT
POSITIONING

MAIN STRUCTURES
VISUALIZED

NOTES

AP ANKLE

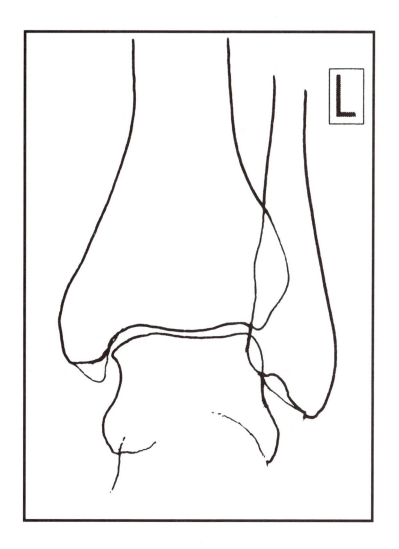

► MEDIAL OBLIQUE ANKLE

CENTERING
LANDMARK AND CR
ORIENTATION

PATIENT
POSITIONING

MAIN STRUCTURES
VISUALIZED

NOTES

MEDIAL OBLIQUE ANKLE

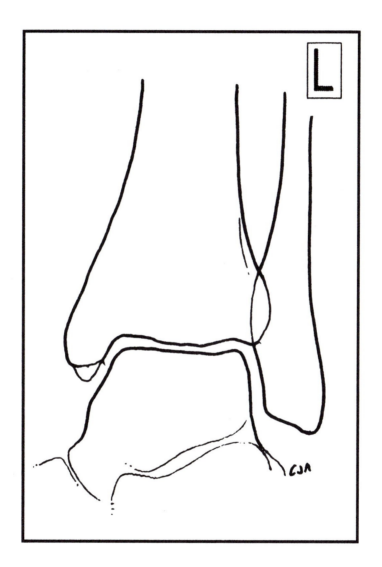

► LATERAL ANKLE

CENTERING
LANDMARK AND CR
ORIENTATION

PATIENT
POSITIONING

MAIN STRUCTURES
VISUALIZED

NOTES

LATERAL ANKLE

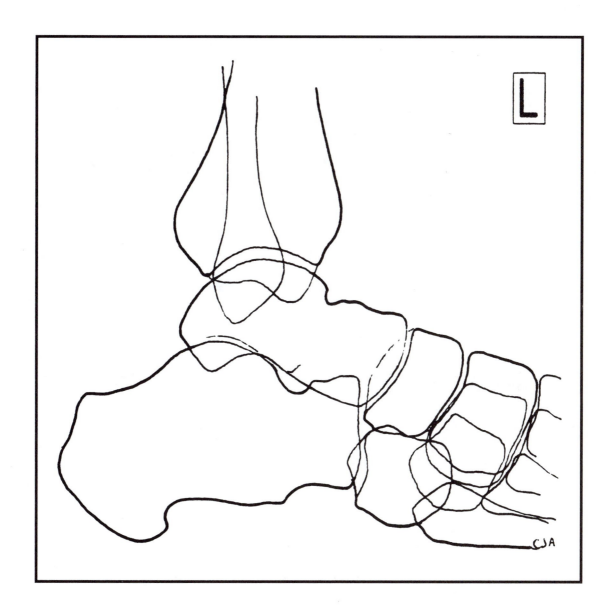

▶ AP LOWER LEG

CENTERING LANDMARK AND CR ORIENTATION

PATIENT POSITIONING

MAIN STRUCTURES VISUALIZED

NOTES

AP LOWER LEG

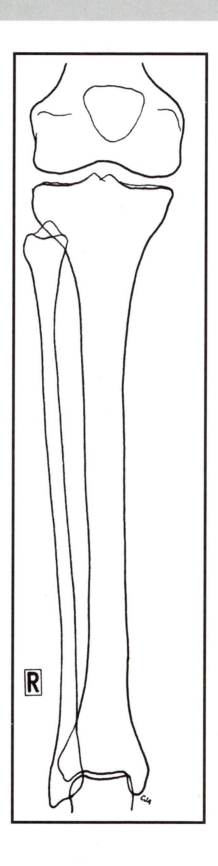

► LATERAL LOWER LEG

CENTERING LANDMARK AND CR ORIENTATION

PATIENT POSITIONING

MAIN STRUCTURES VISUALIZED

NOTES

LATERAL LOWER LEG

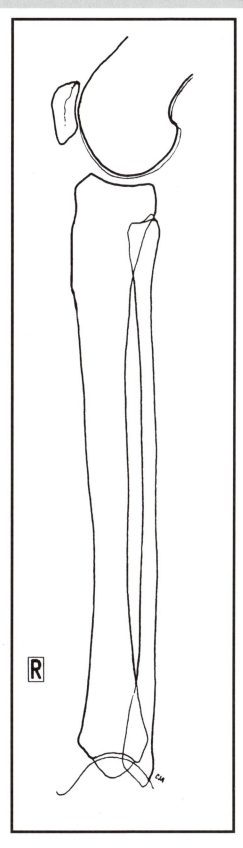

R

▶ AP KNEE

CENTERING LANDMARK AND CR ORIENTATION

PATIENT POSITIONING

MAIN STRUCTURES VISUALIZED

NOTES

AP KNEE

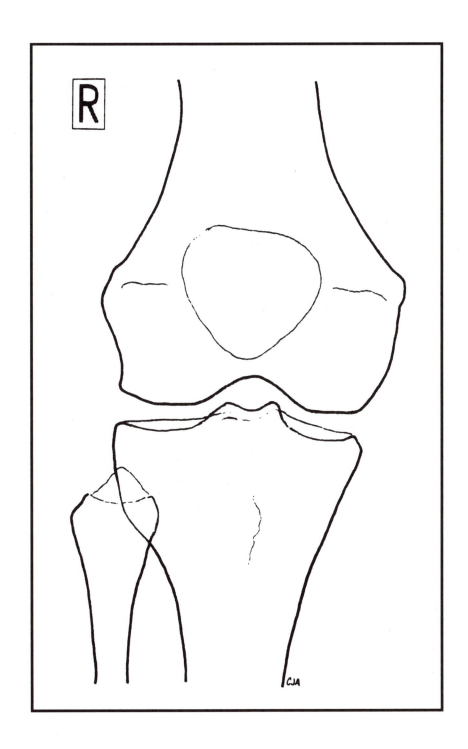

► LATERAL KNEE

CENTERING LANDMARK AND CR ORIENTATION

PATIENT POSITIONING

MAIN STRUCTURES VISUALIZED

NOTES

LATERAL KNEE

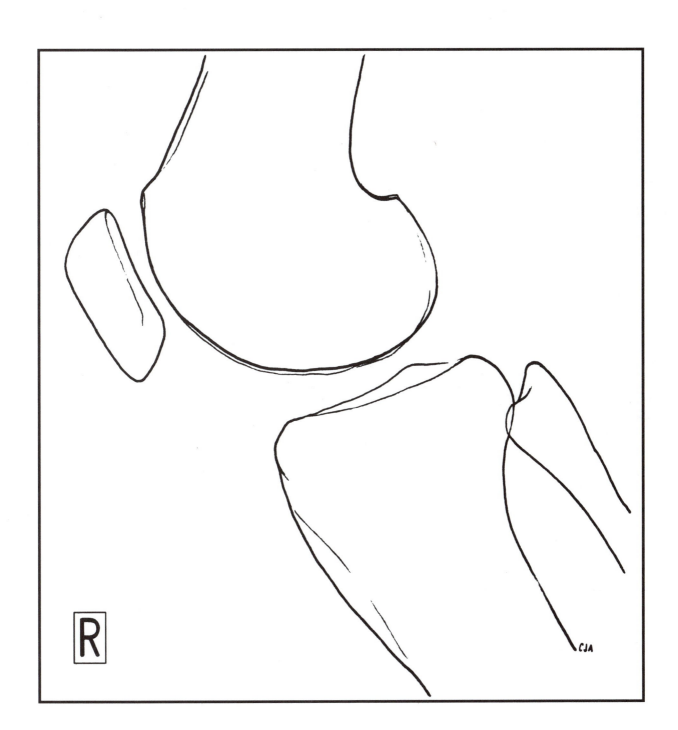

► MEDIAL (INTERNAL) OBLIQUE KNEE

CENTERING LANDMARK AND CR ORIENTATION

PATIENT POSITIONING

MAIN STRUCTURES VISUALIZED

NOTES

MEDIAL (INTERNAL) OBLIQUE KNEE

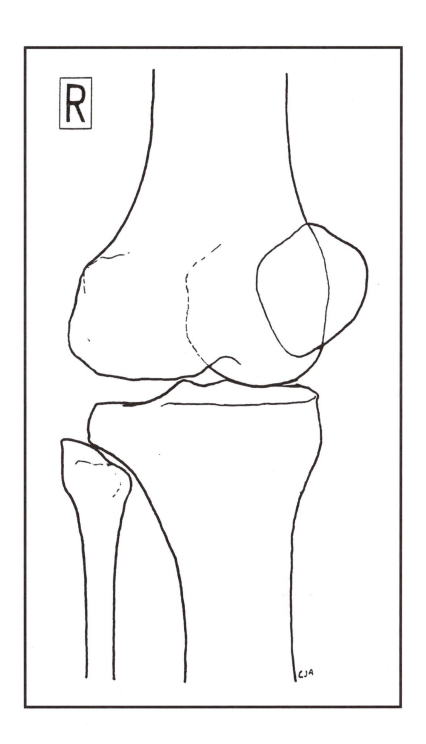

► LATERAL (EXTERNAL) OBLIQUE KNEE

CENTERING LANDMARK AND CR ORIENTATION

PATIENT POSITIONING

MAIN STRUCTURES VISUALIZED

NOTES

LATERAL (EXTERNAL) OBLIQUE KNEE

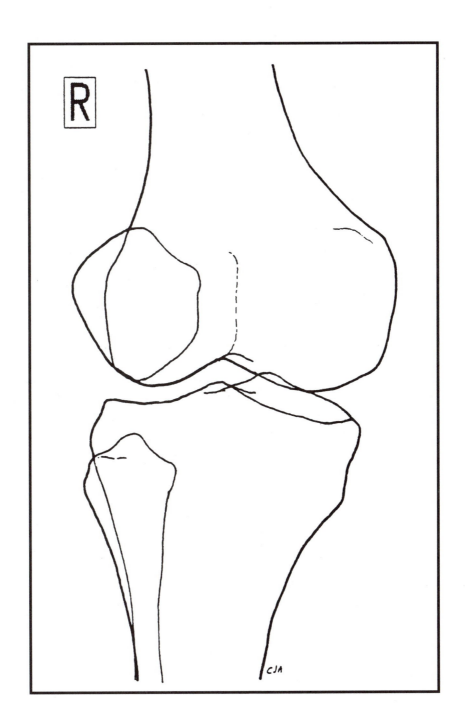

► INTERCONDYLAR FOSSA KNEE

CENTERING
LANDMARK AND CR
ORIENTATION

PATIENT
POSITIONING

MAIN STRUCTURES
VISUALIZED

NOTES

INTERCONDYLAR FOSSA KNEE

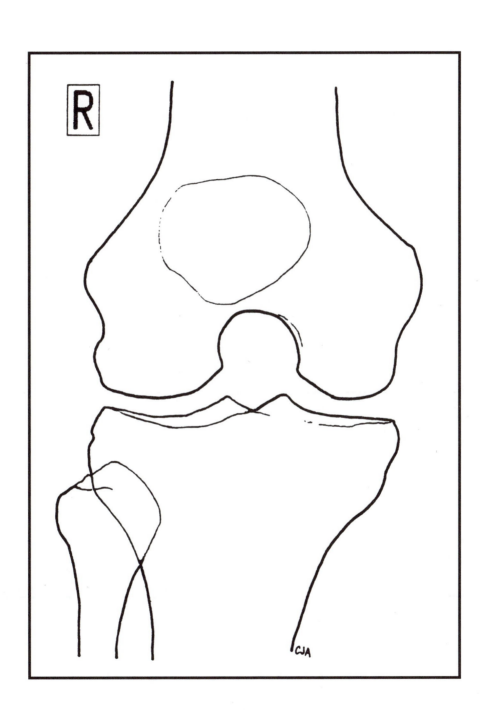

► TANGENTIAL PATELLA

CENTERING
LANDMARK AND CR
ORIENTATION

PATIENT
POSITIONING

MAIN STRUCTURES
VISUALIZED

NOTES

TANGENTIAL PATELLA

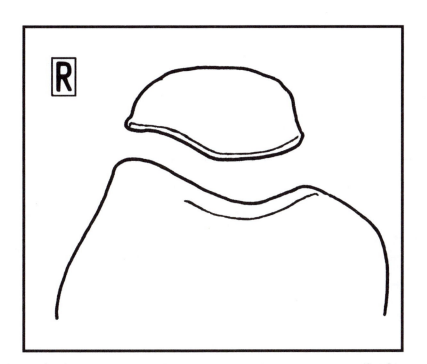

▶ AP FEMUR

CENTERING LANDMARK AND CR ORIENTATION

PATIENT POSITIONING

MAIN STRUCTURES VISUALIZED

NOTES

AP FEMUR

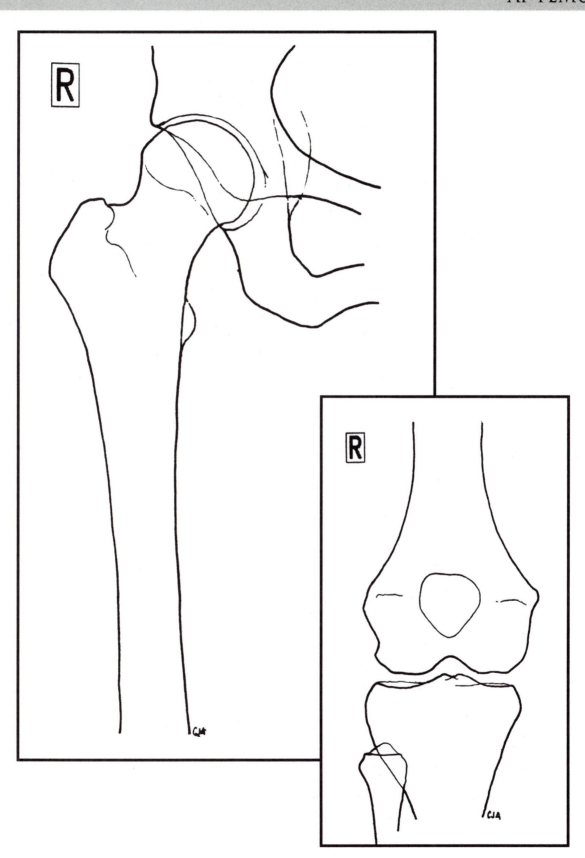

► LATERAL FEMUR

CENTERING LANDMARK AND CR ORIENTATION

PATIENT POSITIONING

MAIN STRUCTURES VISUALIZED

NOTES

LATERAL FEMUR

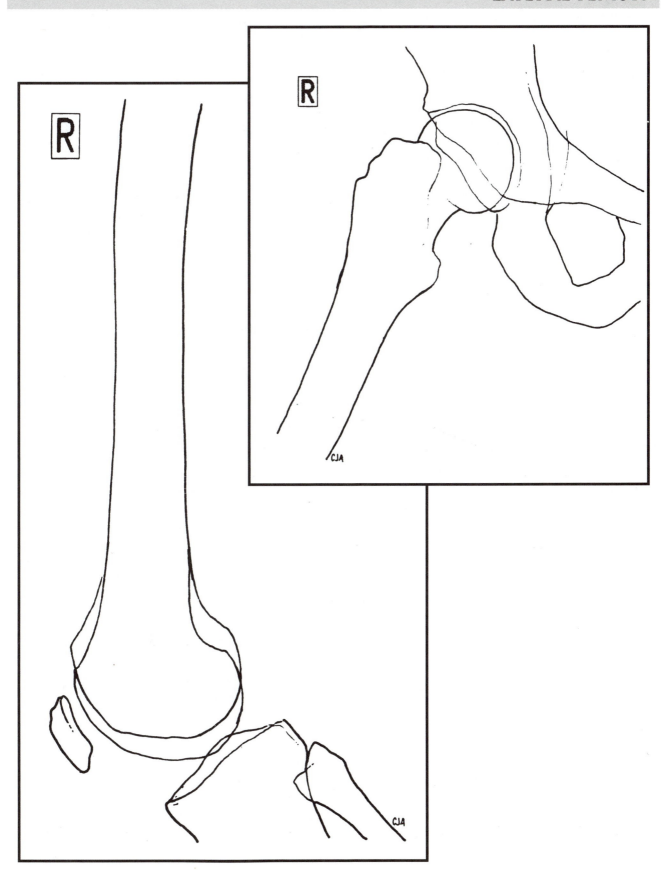

▶ STUDY QUESTIONS

1. How many bones are found in each lower limb? _____

2. The top surface of the foot is called the _____ while the sole or posterior aspect of the foot is the _____ surface.

3. The toes or digits of the foot are comprised of _____ phalanges, which are classified as _____ bones.

4. The great toe (1st digit) is also referred to as the _____ .

5. The heads of the phalanges and metatarsals are located at the _____ (proximal/distal) end of the bone.

6. What part of the metatarsals forms the "ball" of the foot? _____ .

7. The base of which metatarsal is very prominent on the lateral aspect of the foot? _____ .

8. The metatarsals articulate distally with the _____ _____ and proximally with the _____ _____ .

9. Although the metatarsals are similar in structure to the metacarpals of the hand, they are longer and more stout. What is your theory for this difference? _____ _____ _____

10. There are _____ tarsal bones in each foot, which are classified as _____ bones.

11. The _____ cuneiform is also known as the 1st or internal cuneiform.

12. Which tarsal bone articulates proximally with the talus, laterally with the cuboid, and distally with the three cuneiforms? _____

13. The cuboid articulates with which metatarsals? _____ _____ _____

14. The _____ is the largest and strongest tarsal bone.

15. Which tarsal bone(s) is/are involved in the formation of the ankle joint? _____

16. The navicular is also known as the _____ .

17. List the two names of the bone forming the heel of the foot. _____ _____

18. With what bones does the talus articulate? _____ _____

19. Which tarsal bone is also called the astragalus? _____ _____

20. Describe the condition known as *pes planus.* _____ _____

21. The two bones forming the lower leg are the _____ _____ and the _____ . Which of them is/are weight-bearing? _____

22. The calcaneus has _____ articular facets on its upper surface for articulation with the _____ _____ .

23. The shelflike projection of bone on the medial aspect of the calcaneus is called the _____ .

24. What is the purpose of the arches in the foot? _____ _____

25. Which of the bones of the lower leg is located on the medial side of the leg? _____

26. The upper curved area of the talus, which articulates with the tibia, is called the _____ .

27. The sharp ridge of bone that extends down the length of the tibial shaft is the _____ .

28. The large palpable process located on the lateral aspect of the ankle is the _____ . It is located on the _____ (tibia/fibula).

29. Where are the condyles of the tibia located? _____ _____

30. Describe the location and appearance of the tibial plateau. _____
_____

31. The fibula articulates distally with the _____ (head/base) of the tibia at the _____ to form the distal tibiofibular joint.

32. What structure in the lower limb is affected by Osgood–Schlatter disease? _____
_____

33. The head of the fibula is located at the _____ _____ end of the bone.

34. Which bone in the lower limb is considered to be the body's longest and strongest bone? _____

35. Two pointed tubercles that project upward between the articular facets of the tibial plateau are known as the ___ _____ or _____ .

36. The point on the superior aspect of the head of the fibula is known as the _____ or _____ _____ .

37. Name the bones involved in the formation of the knee joint. _____

38. Which bone of the lower limb is considered to be the "calf" bone? _____

39. Describe the location of the fibular notch. _____
_____

40. An injury in which the medial, lateral, and posterior malleoli are fractured is called _____
_____ .

41. The rounded articular structures located on the inferior portion of the femur are the _____ .

42. Where is the tibial tuberosity located? _____
_____

43. Describe the location of the epicondyles of the femur.
_____
_____

44. Name the U-shaped notch on the posterior surface of the femur. _____

45. The femur is not centered in the middle of the thigh but instead lies more _____(anteriorly/ posteriorly) and _____ (medially/ laterally).

46. A vertical ridge of bone called the _____ _____ runs the length of the femoral shaft and serves as the attachment site for the abductor muscles of the thigh.

47. The ligamentum teres extends between the acetabulum of the pelvis and a pit on the femoral head called the _____ to help hold the femur in the socket.

48. A/an _____ is a sesamoid bone that occasionally develops in the muscle behind the lateral condyle of the femur.

49. Which condyle of the femur is larger and extends more distally than the other? _____

50. The head of the femur articulates with the acetabulum on the pelvis to form the hip joint, which has _____ _____ type of movement.

51. The _____ connects the head of the femur to the shaft.

52. The knee cap is formed by a flat triangular bone called the _____ .

53. Of the two prominences situated at the junction of the femoral neck and shaft, the _____ trochanter is located on the lateral margin, while the _____ trochanter is located on the posteromedial aspect of the femur.

54. The lesser and greater trochanters are connected on the posterior aspect of the femur by a ridge of bone called the _____ .

55. The _____ is the flat upper margin of the patella and the pointed inferior surface is called the _____ .

56. What is the only amphiarthrodial joint in the lower limb? _____

57. The first metatarsophalangeal joint is located on the _____ (lateral/medial) side of the foot.

58. What is the "mortise joint" and how can it be demonstrated radiographically? _____ _____

59. Structurally, the distal tibiofibular joint is described as a _____ .

60. The _____ are cartilaginous pads present in the knee joint to cushion the impact of the femur on the tibia.

61. What type of movements are permitted by the knee joint? _____

62. The term *popliteal* refers to _____ _____ .

63. How are the bones that form the knee joint held together as a stable joint? _____ _____

FOR QUESTIONS 64–68 MATCH THE FOLLOWING JOINTS WITH THEIR TYPE OF MOVEMENT.

H = hinge   B = Ball and socket
P = pivot   G = gliding
S = saddle   C = condylar

64. _____ proximal tibiofibular joint

65. _____ intermetatarsal joint between the third and fourth metatarsals

66. _____ interphalangeal joint of the first digit

67. _____ tibiofemoral joint

68. _____ 4th metatarsophalangeal joint

69. Why should the patient remove her shoes prior to radiography of her knee? _____ _____

70. What is the reason for taking weight-bearing AP projections of both knees? _____ _____

71. *Talipes equinovarus* is another name for _____ _____ , which is a congenital deformity involving deviation of the foot from normal alignment.

72. On an AP projection of the foot, the central ray should be directed at an angle of _____ (degree and direction).

73. A medial oblique projection of the toes would be centered at the level of _____ .

74. The foot should be rotated _____ ° (degrees) for a medial oblique projection.

75. What structures would be best demonstrated on the projection described as follows: the patient assumes a position similar to the runner's stance; the foot is dorsiflexed with the plantar surface of the toes resting on the table; the central ray is directed perpendicular to the 1st metatarsophalangeal joint. _____

76. The base of the 5th metatarsal would be best demonstrated on a/an _____ projection of the foot.

77. On which projection of the foot would the plantar surface be positioned perpendicular to the table? _____ _____

78. Indicate the degrees and direction of angulation of the central ray on an axial plantodorsal projection of the calcaneus. _____

79. How do you localize the midpoint of the calcaneus when centering for a lateral projection? _____ _____

80. If a patient fell 10 ft from a ladder and landed directly on his heels, what part of the calcaneus would most likely be injured? _____

81. Why should you have the patient dorsiflex her foot for an AP projection of the ankle? _____ _____

82. If ligament damage is suspected in an ankle injury, what procedure will be performed to assess the extent of the damage? _____ _____

83. How do you locate the ankle joint for centering purposes by using the malleoli as landmarks?_____

_____

84. What is the recommended kVp for a radiographic examination of the lower leg? Is a grid or screen technique used?_____

85. You are evaluating a lateral projection of the lower leg for accurate positioning. Describe the relationship of the tibia and fibula._____

_____

86. Which projection of the knee will best demonstrate the tibial plateau and intercondylar eminence?_____

_____

87. The _____ projection of the lower leg will best demonstrate the tibial tuberosity in profile.

88. How many degrees and in what direction should the central ray be directed for an AP projection of the knee? Explain the need for the angle._____

_____

89. How many degrees must the knee be rotated for medial (internal) and lateral (external) oblique projections?

_____

90. Which projection of the knee will demonstrate the patella partially superimposed over the lateral femoral condyle?_____

91. Why is it recommended that the central ray be angled _____ (degree and direction) on a lateral projection of the knee? _____

_____

92. List the routine projections for radiography of the lower leg:_____

93. On a lateral projection of the knee, the joint should be flexed approximately _____ ° (degrees).

94. The femoral condyles are superimposed on the _____ projection of the femur.

95. On a PA axial projection of the intercondylar fossa, the central ray is directed _____ to the long axis of the tibia.

96. To maximize the femoropatellar joint space and minimize the chance of separating fracture fragments when taking a lateral projection of the patella, the knee should be flexed _____ ° (degrees).

97. When radiographing the intercondylar fossa, you prefer to use the Holmblad method, which entails having the patient kneel on the table and directing the CR perpendicular to the knee. However, your patient is an elderly gentleman who is unable to kneel on the table. Describe how you will achieve the desired radiograph using an alternative method._____

_____

_____

98. Explain the reason why an AP projection of the knee or a PA projection of the patella should be taken prior to taking a sunrise projection of the patella._____

_____

99. You are taking a tangential (sunrise) projection of the patella. Your patient is lying prone on the table with his knee flexed at an angle slightly less than 90°. How many degrees and in what direction must you angle the central ray?_____

100. A radiographic examination of the femur has been ordered on a very tall man. How will you determine if the knee joint or hip joint should be included on the film?

_____

_____

101. Why should the entire leg be rotated 5° internally for an AP projection of the femur?_____

_____

102. Describe the position of the right leg when you are taking a lateral projection of the left distal femur._____

_____

103. What is the purpose of a *scanogram*?_____

_____

_____

104. Complete the following table:

Projection	CR Angle/Angle of Part	Centering Point	Film Size	Structures Seen
Lateral foot				
Medial (internal) oblique knee				
PA patella				
PA axial intercondylar fossa (Camp Coventry method)				
AP femur				

► CASE STUDIES

1. While running through a field of high grass, a 10-year-old boy suddenly feels a sharp pain in his left foot. Upon inspection, he sees that he has stepped on a nail, which was sticking up through an old board. The nail is very long, has punctured the sole of his tennis shoe, and is projecting through the top of his foot. The boy is transported to the hospital with a 4 × 10-in. plank of board attached to his foot. The radiographic request calls for a foot series.

   ► Since the shoe and board can not be removed prior to radiography, what type of artifact will they leave on the radiograph? How will the nail appear?

   ► Discuss the method you will use to obtain projections of the foot with the board attached. Will you angle on the AP projection? Explain your answer.

   ► Explain why you were asked to radiograph the patient's foot *before* the board and nail were removed.

2. A 40-year-old woman dropped a large can of fruit on her right foot. Because her foot was swollen and painful, her physician sent her to the outpatient department for radiographs. Due to severe rheumatoid arthritis in her knees, the patient is unable to bend her right knee sufficiently to place the plantar surface of the foot flat on the table.

   ► Describe how you would obtain the three-view foot series that has been requested.

3. A 25-year-old male is transported to the emergency department by ambulance following a hiking accident in which his right lower leg was crushed by a large boulder. The leg is encased in an air splint. You are requested to take radiographs of the lower leg to include both joints. The ER physician explains that it is very important to include the entire tibia, fibula, and both joints on the same film. The entire leg will not fit on a 7 × 17-in. cassette oriented lengthwise, which is the usual protocol.

   ▸ Describe how you will successfully complete the radiographic examination.

   ▸ Should the air splint be removed prior to radiography? If not, how will it visualize on the radiographs?

4. Your patient is a 36-year-old female who gave you a history of being hit directly in the left kneecap by a log while stacking firewood. She is unable to straighten her leg for radiographs of the knee.

   ▸ What possible injuries might she have sustained?

   ▸ If the patella is injured, what projection(s) will best demonstrate the pathology?

   ▸ Should you attempt to straighten the patient's leg? Explain your answer.

5. Your patient is a developmentally disabled teenager who normally is in the fetal position. He fell out of bed and his right knee has become swollen and bruised. He is sent to the imaging department for a "four-view" radiographic examination of the knee, which includes AP knee, lateral knee, tangential patella, and intercondylar fossa. The patient's leg can be straightened for short periods of time if it is immobilized; otherwise, it must be held for the examination.

   ▸ Describe how you would achieve AP and lateral projections of the knee.

   ▸ Discuss the methods you will use to obtain the tangential projection of the patella and the projection of the intercondylar fossa.

6. A 45-year-old male was using a power nailer to put shingles on a roof when he felt himself slipping off the roof. When he tried to catch himself, he accidentally put a nail into his thigh just proximal to the knee. The pain of the injury caused him to fall off the roof, resulting in an injury to his neck and lower back. He was transported to the emergency department on a backboard. Radiographs of his cervical and lumbar spine were ordered, along with AP and lateral projections of the femur for foreign body.

▸ Discuss how you would proceed with this case. Which radiograph will you take first?

▸ What considerations would affect positioning for the remaining radiographs?

▸ In what order would you take the remaining radiographs?

► POSITIONING WORKSHEETS

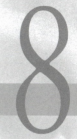

COLOR EACH BONE ONE COLOR AND LABEL THE FOLLOWING ANATOMIC PARTS ON THE DRAWINGS FOR THIS SECTION. LABEL ALL PARTS THAT CAN BE SEEN ON EACH POSITION OR PROJECTION.

PELVIS: AP

- ► ILIUM
  - Ala
  - Crest of ilium
- ► ISCHIUM
  - Ischial tuberosity

- ► PUBIS
- ► ACETABULUM
- ► OBTURATOR FORAMEN
- ► SACRUM
- ► L5

- ► FEMUR
  - Head
  - Neck
  - Greater trochanter

- ► ARTICULATIONS
  - Hip
  - Sacroiliac
  - Symphysis pubis

HIP: AP Oblique (Frogleg), Transfemoral Lateral

- ► PELVIS
  - Ilium
  - Acetabulum

- Obturator foramen
- Ischial tuberosity

- ► FEMUR
  - Head
  - Neck

- Greater trochanter
- Lesser trochanter

SACROILIAC JOINTS: AP Obliques

- ► ILIUM
- ► SACRUM
- ► L5
- ► SI ARTICULATION

COMPLETE THE APPROPRIATE INFORMATION SHEET FOR EACH DRAWING.

8

PELVIC GIRDLE

► AP PELVIS

CENTERING LANDMARK AND CR ORIENTATION

PATIENT POSITIONING

MAIN STRUCTURES VISUALIZED

NOTES

AP PELVIS

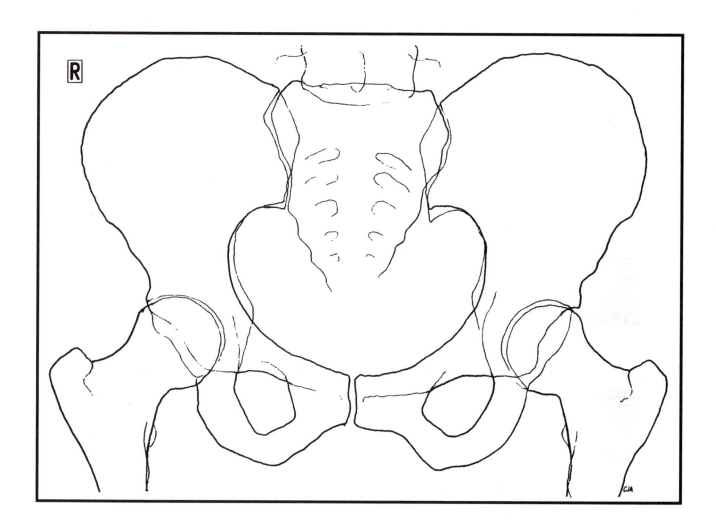

► AP OBLIQUE (FROGLEG) HIP

CENTERING LANDMARK AND CR ORIENTATION

....
....
....
....
....
....

PATIENT POSITIONING

....
....
....
....
....

MAIN STRUCTURES VISUALIZED

....
....
....
....
....

NOTES

....
....
....
....
....
....

AP OBLIQUE (FROGLEG) HIP

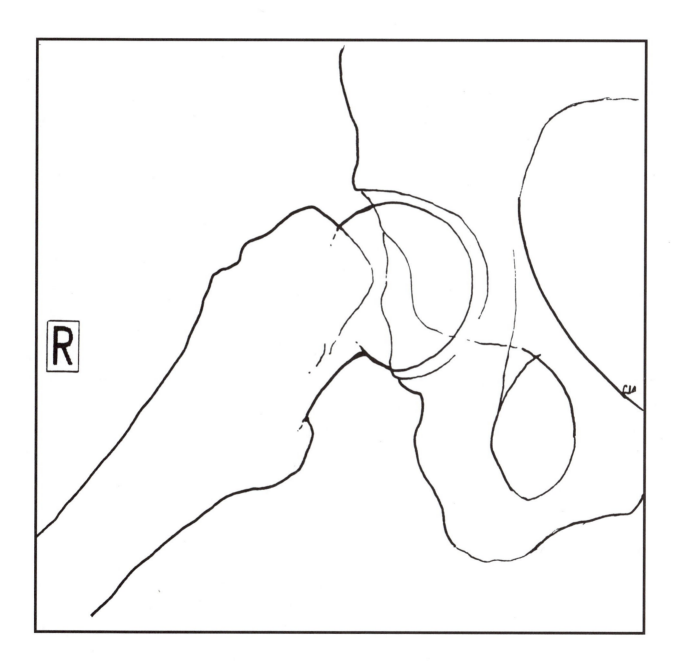

▶ TRANSFEMORAL LATERAL HIP

CENTERING
LANDMARK AND CR
ORIENTATION

PATIENT
POSITIONING

MAIN STRUCTURES
VISUALIZED

NOTES

TRANSFEMORAL LATERAL HIP

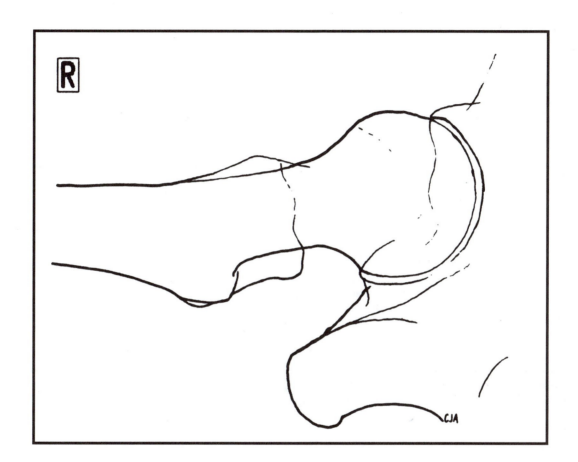

► AP OBLIQUE SACROILIAC JOINTS

CENTERING LANDMARK AND CR ORIENTATION

PATIENT POSITIONING

MAIN STRUCTURES VISUALIZED

NOTES

► LPO   AP OBLIQUE SACROILIAC JOINTS   ► RPO

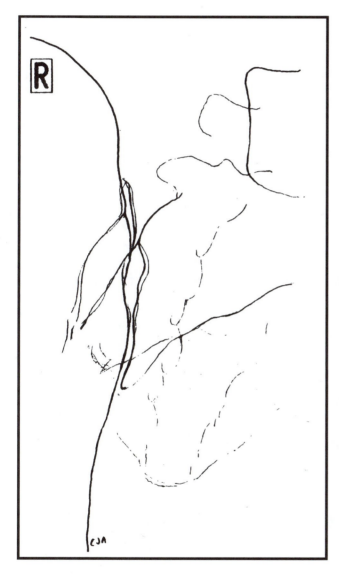

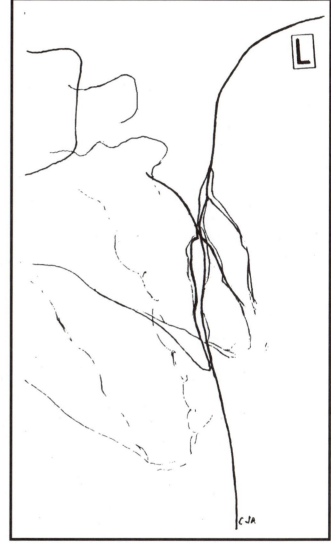

▶ STUDY QUESTIONS

1. The "hip bones" are formed by the _____ _____ or _____ .

2. The three bones forming each hip bone are the _____ _____ .

3. List two functions of the pelvic girdle. _____ _____

4. The deep cup-shaped depression on either lower lateral margin of the pelvis is the _____ .

5. Name the L-shaped bone that forms the posteroinferior portion of the hip bone. _____

6. The _____ is the largest division of the hip bone and is located superior to the acetabulum.

7. The _____ forms the anteroinferior aspect of the hip bone.

8. The ilium, ischium, and pubis fuse with one another at the _____ .

9. Which of the bones of the pelvic girdle is described as a V-shaped bone consisting of a body and two rami? _____

10. The _____ is the upper flared portion of the ilium.

11. Where is the iliac fossa located? _____ _____

12. The _____ is a palpable bony landmark situated at the anterior end of the iliac crest.

13. A deep indentation on the posterior aspect of the ilium between the posterior inferior iliac spine (PIIS) and ischial spine is the _____ .

14. The curved upper margin of the ala of the ilium is called the _____ .

15. Where is the body of the ilium located? _____ _____

16. On which bone is the lesser sciatic notch located? _____ _____

17. The _____ is the ear-shaped area on the ilium that articulates with the sacrum to form the sacroiliac joint.

18. The _____ is a rounded, roughened process on the inferior aspect of the pelvis that supports the weight of a person when he/she sits.

19. The _____ of the ischium extends from the body to join the pubis.

20. The gluteal lines on the _____ surface of the ilium serve as the attachment site for the gluteal muscles.

21. The ilium forms the upper _____ (ratio) of the acetabulum.

22. The lower, posterior _____ (ratio) of the acetabulum is formed by the ischium.

23. The pubis forms the anterior _____ (ratio) of the acetabulum.

24. The _____ of the right and left pubic bones meet at the midline of the body to form the symphysis pubis.

25. The _____ of the pubis extends inferiorly from the symphysis pubis to join the ramus of the ischium.

26. The rami of the ischium and pubis form a bony loop that encircles an opening known as the _____ .

27. Where is the pubic arch located? _____ _____

28. A triangular bony structure on the ischium that projects posteriorly from the acetabulum and medially into the pelvic cavity is the _____ .

29. The _____ is a small ridge of bone on the anterior border of the superior ramus of the pubis.

30. The superior ramus of the pubis extends _____ (laterally/medially) from the acetabulum.

31. The _____ (false/true) pelvis is located above the pelvic brim.

32. The pelvic brim is a bony ridge passing obliquely from the _____ to the _____ _____ .

33. Where is the ischial spine located in relationship to the greater sciatic notch? _____ _____

34. The pelvic brim is also known as the _____ _____ as it forms the upper border of the pelvic cavity.

35. The uterus, urinary bladder, and rectum of a female are located within the _____ (false/true) pelvis.

36. The pelvic outlet is bounded anteriorly by the _____ _____ , posteriorly by the _____ _____ , and laterally by the _____ _____ .

37. The _____ (false/true) pelvis supports the abdominal organs as well as the developing fetus during pregnancy.

38. The true pelvis is also known as the _____ _____ (greater/lesser) pelvis, and the false pelvis is also called the _____ (greater/lesser) pelvis.

39. The ilia of the _____ (female/male) pelvis are described as broader, less curved, and more shallow than those of the opposite sex.

40. How does the appearance of the pubic arch differ between male and female pelves? _____ _____

41. What type of examination is currently performed during pregnancy to measure the inlet and outlet of the maternal pelvis as well as the head of the fetus? _____ _____

42. What two structures articulate to form the hip joint? ____ _____

43. What is a "coxal" joint? _____ _____

44. Which joints of the pelvic girdle are described as wedge-shaped? _____

45. Structurally, the symphysis pubis is _____ _____ and is classified according to function (movement) as _____ .

46. Explain why the acetabulum is considered initially to be a synchondrosis and then a synostosis. _____ _____

47. The hip joint is classified according to structure as _____ _____ .

48. How is the hip joint classified according to function (movement)? _____ _____

49. What is the functional (movement) classification of the sacroiliac (S-I) joints? _____ _____

50. What is Legg–Calve–Perthes disease? _____ _____

51. Why should the radiographer question the patient about previous hip surgery prior to radiography of the hip? ____ _____

52. Why should the legs be internally rotated 15–20° for an AP projection of the pelvis? _____ _____

53. Why is internal rotation of the legs contraindicated when a fracture of the proximal femur is suspected? _____ _____

54. Describe the appearance of the lesser trochanters of the femurs when the legs are internally rotated. _____ _____

55. Describe how the femoral neck can be localized for radiography of the hip. _____ _____

56. AP and lateral projections of the hip are ordered on a patient with a suspected fracture of the femoral neck. What method will you use to obtain the lateral projection? _____ _____

57. Why must the patient be obliqued to adequately demonstrate the sacroiliac (S-I) joints? _____ _____

58. The patient must be rotated approximately _____ ° (degrees) to an RPO or LPO position to demonstrate the S-I joints.

59. If the patient is in an RPO position, the _____ (right/left) S-I joint will be best demonstrated.

60. The central ray must be angled _____ (degree and direction) on a PA axial projection of the S-I joints.

61. How will rotation be demonstrated on an AP projection of the pelvis? _____ _____

62. For the AP oblique (frogleg) projection of the hip, the patient's hip and knee should be flexed and the leg abducted _____ ° (degrees).

63. Approximately how much of the proximal femur should be included on an AP or lateral projection of the hip? _____ _____

64. On a transfemoral lateral projection of the hip, the central ray should be directed _____ (parallel/perpendicular) to the femoral neck.

65. Your patient is unable to lie on her abdomen for the PA axial projection of the S-I joints. What can you do to achieve a radiograph demonstrating the same anatomy? _____ _____

66. On an AP axial projection of the anterior pelvic bones, the central ray should be directed _____ (degree and direction) for a female patient and _____ _____ (degree and direction) for a male patient. Explain why there is a difference in the degree of angulation. _____ _____

67. Describe the appearance of the rami of the ischia and pubis on the superoinferior axial projection of the anterior pelvic bones (Lilienfeld method). _____ _____

68. An AP oblique projection of the acetabulum (Judet method) requires the patient to be positioned in a _____ ° (degrees) oblique with the affected hip elevated from the table.

69. On the PA axial oblique projection of the acetabulum (Teufel method), the central ray should be directed _____ _____ (degree and direction) through the hip joint at the level of the _____ .

INDICATE TRUE OR FALSE FOR QUESTIONS 70-74.

_____ 70. In addition to allowing for the passage of nerves and blood vessels, the obturator foramina serve to lessen the weight of the pelvis.

_____ 71. The ilium, ischium, and pubis form a bony ring around the obturator foramen.

_____ 72. The sacrum tends to be longer and more curved on a female pelvis, resulting in a longer, more curved pelvic cavity.

_____ 73. Although the hip and shoulder joints are similarly classified according to movement, the movement of the hip joint is limited by the depth of the acetabulum.

_____ 74. On an AP axial projection of the pelvic outlet, the rami of the pubis and ischia should appear elongated or "stretched out" with no superimposition evident.

75. Complete the following table:

Projection	CR Angle/Angle of Part	Centering Point	Film Size	Structures Seen
AP pelvis				
AP oblique (frogleg) hip (mod. Cleaves)				
Lateral hip (Lauenstein method)				
LPO for S-I joints				
AP oblique acetabulum (Judet method)				

▶ CASE STUDIES

1. While walking across the street, a 65-year-old woman was struck by a bicycle. She has sustained injuries to her left hip and ankle, and is transported to radiology by stretcher. The requisition states that there are possible fractures of the hip and ankle, and radiographic examinations of the hip and ankle have been ordered. When you examine the patient, you see that her left foot is turned outward and the left leg is bent, appearing slightly shorter than the right leg. This leads you to believe that the hip is indeed fractured and you must proceed with extreme caution.

   ▶ How is the appearance of the patient's leg indicative of a fracture?

   ▶ Explain how you would radiograph her hip without moving her leg.

   ▶ Identify the two projections that should be taken to demonstrate a hip fracture.

   ▶ Describe how you would achieve the standard three-view ankle radiographs without changing the position of the patient's leg.

2. A very tall 20-year-old male is brought to the imaging department following a motorcycle accident. Since the injury is to the proximal third of the femur, radiographs of the hip and femur have been ordered. Due to the type of injury, the patient is unable to abduct his leg into the frogleg position.

   ▶ Discuss the method you will use to take two projections of the hip.

   ▶ Describe how you will take the AP and lateral projections of the femur, including centering point, film orientation, and positioning.

....

....

....

....

....

....

....

....

....

....

3. Your patient sustained multiple lacerations to her lower back and is complaining of severe pain in the area of her right S-I joint. A radiographic examination of the S-I joints has been ordered. The routine series normally consists of AP axial and bilateral oblique projections of the S-I joints; however, the patient is unable to roll into a posterior oblique or supine position for the traditional radiographs.

   ▶ Describe how you would obtain oblique projections of the S-I joints.

   ▶ Explain how you must modify the axial projection of the S-I joints since the patient is in the prone position.

....

....

....

....

....

....

....

....

....

....

....

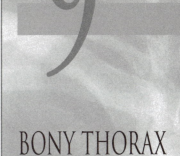

▶ POSITIONING WORKSHEETS

COLOR EACH BONE OR TYPE OF BONE ONE COLOR AND LA-
BEL THE FOLLOWING ANATOMICAL PARTS ON THE DRAWINGS
FOR THIS SECTION. LABEL ALL PARTS THAT CAN BE SEEN ON
EACH POSITION OR PROJECTION.

STERNUM: RAO, Lateral

▶ STERNUM	Body	▶ THORACIC SPINE	Sternocostal
Jugular notch	Xiphoid process	▶ ARTICULATIONS	Costovertebral
Manubrium	▶ CLAVICLE	S-C joint	
Sternal angle	▶ RIBS		

S-C JOINTS: PA, Oblique

▶ STERNUM	Manubrium	▶ CLAVICLE	▶ THORACIC SPINE
Jugular notch	Sternal angle	▶ RIBS	▶ S-C ARTICULATION

RIBS: AP/PA, Oblique

▶ RIBS	▶ CLAVICLE	▶ THORACIC SPINE	▶ DIAPHRAGM
Number 1 through 12			

COMPLETE THE APPROPRIATE INFORMATION SHEET FOR
EACH DRAWING.

9

BONY THORAX

► RAO STERNUM

CENTERING
LANDMARK AND CR
ORIENTATION

PATIENT
POSITIONING

MAIN STRUCTURES
VISUALIZED

NOTES

RAO STERNUM

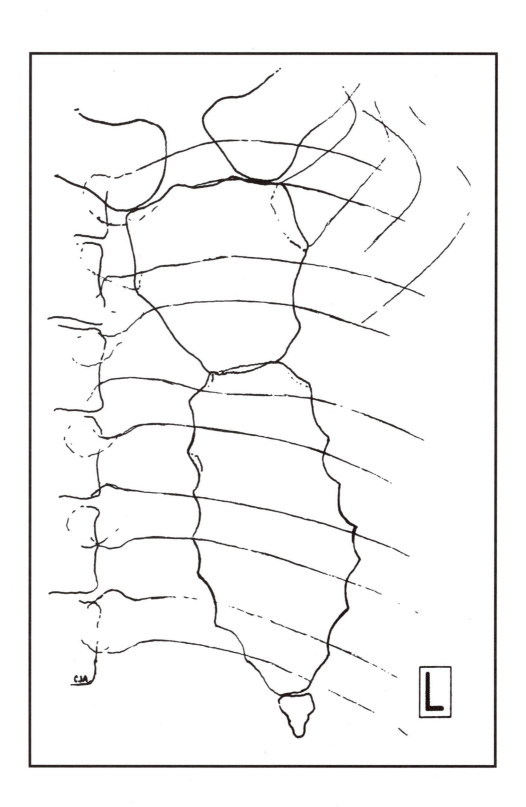

► LATERAL STERNUM

CENTERING
LANDMARK AND CR
ORIENTATION

PATIENT
POSITIONING

MAIN STRUCTURES
VISUALIZED

NOTES

LATERAL STERNUM

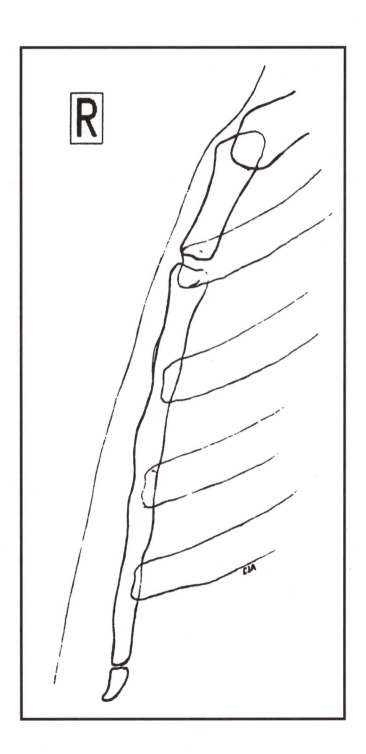

► PA STERNOCLAVICULAR JOINTS

CENTERING LANDMARK AND CR ORIENTATION

PATIENT POSITIONING

MAIN STRUCTURES VISUALIZED

NOTES

PA STERNOCLAVICULAR JOINTS

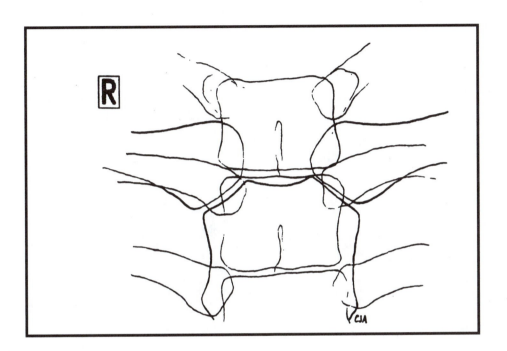

▶ PA OBLIQUE STERNOCLAVICULAR JOINTS

CENTERING LANDMARK AND CR ORIENTATION

PATIENT POSITIONING

MAIN STRUCTURES VISUALIZED

NOTES

PA OBLIQUE STERNOCLAVICULAR JOINTS

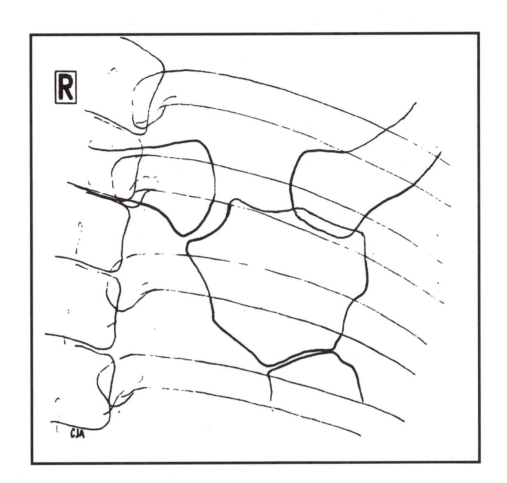

▶ AP RIBS (ABOVE THE DIAPHRAGM)

CENTERING
LANDMARK AND CR
ORIENTATION

PATIENT
POSITIONING

MAIN STRUCTURES
VISUALIZED

NOTES

AP RIBS (ABOVE THE DIAPHRAGM)

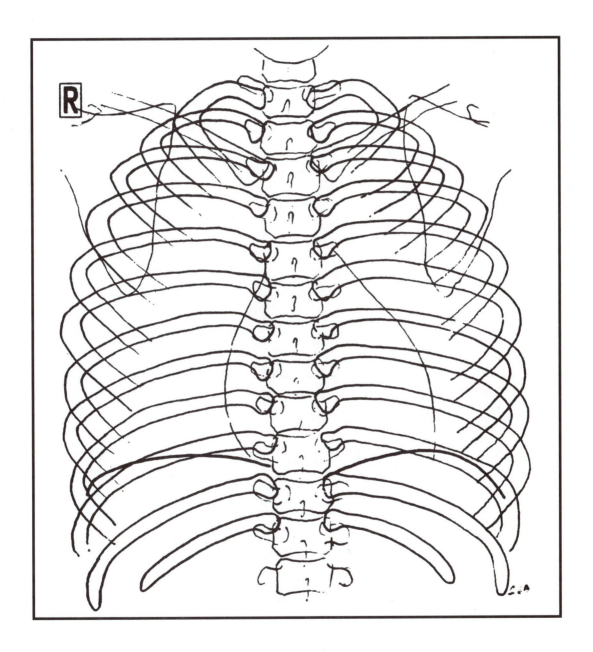

► AP RIBS (BELOW THE DIAPHRAGM)

CENTERING LANDMARK AND CR ORIENTATION

PATIENT POSITIONING

MAIN STRUCTURES VISUALIZED

NOTES

AP RIBS (BELOW THE DIAPHRAGM)

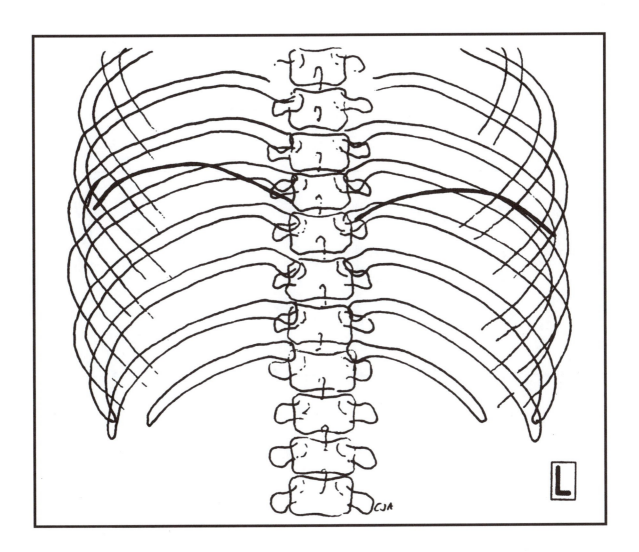

▶ OBLIQUE RIBS

CENTERING
LANDMARK AND CR
ORIENTATION

PATIENT
POSITIONING

MAIN STRUCTURES
VISUALIZED

NOTES

OBLIQUE RIBS

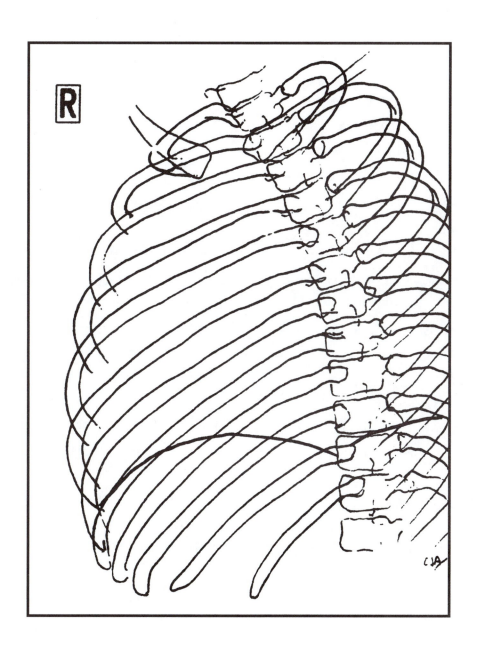

▶ STUDY QUESTIONS

1. List the bones that constitute the bony thorax. _____

   _____

2. Explain how the bony thorax forms a "cage" that surrounds and protects the organs of the thoracic cavity. ____

   _____

   _____

3. Which bone of the bony thorax forms the *breastbone?*

   _____

4. There are _____ pairs of ribs in the bony thorax.

5. The ribs are classified as what type of bones? _____

   _____

6. The two ends of the ribs are known as the _____

   and _____ends or extremities.

7. The head and neck of the rib is located at the bone's ____

   _____ (anterior/posterior) end.

8. A small bump located on the dorsal surface of the rib between the neck and shaft is the _____ .

9. The _____ of the rib is the point at which the shaft curves forward.

10. Blood vessels and nerves are housed in the _____

    _____ on the inner curved surface of the shaft of the rib.

11. Where is the costal cartilage located? _____

    _____

12. What part of the rib articulates with a thoracic vertebra?

    _____

13. The _____ space is located between adjacent ribs.

14. The _____ extremity is located at the anterior end of the rib.

15. True ribs are also known as _____ ribs.

16. Which ribs are considered to be true ribs? Explain why.

    _____

    _____

17. False ribs are also known as _____ ribs.

18. Which pairs of ribs are designated as false ribs? _____

    _____

19. What forms the *costal arch?* _____

    _____

20. Which pairs of ribs are called *floating* or *vertebral* ribs?

    _____

21. The _____ through _____ ribs articulate with two adjacent thoracic vertebrae, while the _____ ribs articulate with the correspondingly numbered vertebral bodies.

22. Why do rib fractures usually result in extreme pain and bruising at the site of the injury? _____

    _____

23. How do the intercostal muscles function during respiration? _____

    _____

24. How is the costal cartilage demonstrated on a PA projection of the upper ribs? _____

    _____

25. List the three divisions of the sternum. _____

    _____

26. The sternum is classified as a/an _____ bone.

27. The most superior portion of the sternum is the _____

    _____ .

28. _____ is another name for the body of the sternum.

29. The inferior tip of the sternum is the _____

    _____ .

30. The juncture between the manubrium and the body of the sternum is called the _____

31. The diaphragm attaches to which part of the sternum? _____

32. Why are compressions during CPR *never* performed over the xiphoid process? _____ _____

33. *Cost/o-* means _____ and *chondr/o-* means _____ .

34. Relative to the spine, the sternal angle corresponds to the level of _____ .

35. Another name for the xiphoid process is the _____ _____ .

36. Discuss how the sternum is occasionally used in bone marrow transplantations. _____ _____

37. The _____ is a slight depression that is palpable on the superior border of the sternum. It is also known as the _____ .

38. Relative to the spine, the xiphoid process corresponds to the level of _____ .

39. Relative to the spine, the jugular notch corresponds to the level of _____ .

40. The first pair of ribs articulates with the _____ _____ of the sternum.

41. Describe the location of the clavicular notches on the sternum. _____ _____

42. What is a "facet"? _____ _____

43. What is the "S-C" joint? _____ _____

44. The xiphoid process generally ossifies and fuses to the sternal body around the age of _____ .

45. The _____ joint on the sternum corresponds to the sternal angle.

46. How does the 1st sternocostal joint differ from the 2nd through 7th sternocostal joints with regard to structure and function? _____ _____

47. What structures articulate to form the costochondral joints? _____ _____

48. The articulation of the head of a rib with a thoracic vertebra forms the _____ joint, while the articulation of the tubercle with the transverse process of the vertebra forms the _____ joint.

49. The sternoclavicular joints are classified according to structure as _____ and function (movement) as _____ .

50. To demonstrate the axillary portion of the left ribs, the patient should be placed in either the _____ or _____ position.

51. To demonstrate the heads and necks of the left ribs, the patient should be placed in either the _____ _____ or _____ position.

52. Why is the RAO position preferred over the LAO for radiography of the sternum? _____ _____

53. The patient is normally rotated _____ ° (degrees) for the RAO position of the sternum.

54. Larger patients must be rotated _____ (more/less) than thinner patients to project the sternum free from superimposition over the spine.

55. To demonstrate the sternoclavicular joints, the patient must be rotated _____ ° (degrees) from the prone position.

56. What projection will best demonstrate the left sternoclavicular joint? _____

57. What is the purpose of using a long exposure time for the RAO position of the sternum? _____ _____

58. What breathing instructions should be given to the patient for an AP projection of the ribs below the diaphragm? _____

59. Why should a 72-in. SID be used whenever possible for the lateral projection of the sternum? _____ _____

60. What is the advantage of using a 30-in. SID instead of the 40-in. for the RAO position of the sternum? _____ _____

61. How many ribs should be included on an AP or PA projection of the ribs above the diaphragm? _____ _____

62. How many ribs should be included on an AP or PA projection of the ribs below the diaphragm? _____ _____

63. Why is a relatively low kVp setting of 60–65 kVp recommended for radiography of the ribs above the diaphragm? _____ _____

64. On the PA oblique (RAO) projection of the sternum, the central ray should be directed to the midpoint of the sternum at the level of _____ .

65. As you are viewing a PA oblique (RAO) projection of the sternum, you note that the manubrium is superimposed over the vertebral column. How will you correct this positioning error? _____ _____

66. What breathing instructions are given to the patient for a lateral projection of the sternum? _____ _____

67. The sternoclavicular joint _____ (farthest/nearest) the film will be best demonstrated on PA oblique projections.

68. Why should the patient place his hands behind his back for the lateral projection of the sternum? _____ _____

69. Why is it recommended that the patient raise her arms over her head for the AP projection of the ribs above the diaphragm? _____ _____

INDICATE TRUE OR FALSE FOR QUESTIONS 70–74.

_____ 70. Radiography of the ribs should be performed in the recumbent position because it is easier for the patient to maintain the position when in pain.

_____ 71. Of the articulations formed by the bones of the bony thorax, no single joint permits more than gliding movement.

_____ 72. The second pair of ribs articulates with the sternum at the level of the sternal angle.

_____ 73. The xiphoid process is generally the longest part of the sternum.

_____ 74. Because the distance between the spine and sternum is less on thinner patients than on larger patients, thinner patients must be rotated more to adequately demonstrate the sternoclavicular joints.

75. Complete the following table:

Projection	CR Angle/Angle of Part	Centering Point	Film Size	Structures Seen
Lateral sternum				
RAO S-C joints				
RPO ribs				
PA ribs below the diaphragm				

► CASE STUDIES

1. A 60-year-old male is experiencing severe sternal pain several days following heart surgery. He is brought to the radiology department on a stretcher for radiographic examination of his sternum. Due to his surgical incision, he is unable to roll into an anterior oblique or prone position.

   ► Describe how you will obtain the two radiographs of the sternum with the patient in a supine or posterior oblique position.

   ► What effect will this modification in positioning have on the radiographic appearance of the sternum?

   ► If the patient is unable to sit erect, how will you obtain the lateral projection?

2. A patient has been brought in from the local jail because he is complaining of painful breathing after being arrested for fighting. Radiographic examination of the right and left ribs is ordered. The patient's hands and feet are shackled to the stretcher and the accompanying police officer is reluctant to unlock the restraints.

   ► Given the patient's limited mobility, discuss the method you will use to obtain the necessary radiographs of his ribs.

▶ POSITIONING WORKSHEETS

COLOR EACH BONE OR TYPE OF BONE (IE, LUMBAR VERTE-
BREA) ONE COLOR AND LABEL THE FOLLOWING ANATOMIC
PARTS ON THE DRAWINGS FOR THIS SECTION. LABEL ALL
PARTS THAT CAN BE SEEN ON EACH POSITION OR PROJEC-
TION.

CERVICAL SPINE: AP, Oblique, Lateral, AP Atlas and Axis

▶ CERVICAL VERTEBRAE	Transverse process	Vertebra prominens	▶ ARTICULATIONS
C1–7	Body	Dens	Intervertebral disk space
Pedicle	Intervertebral foramina	Lateral mass of C-1	Zygapophyseal joint
Spinous process	Articular pillar		

THORACIC SPINE: AP, Lateral, Lateral Cervicothoracic Region

▶ THORACIC VERTEBRAE	Transverse process	▶ CLAVICLE	Intervertebral disk space
T1–12	Body	▶ RIBS 1–12	Costovertebral
Pedicle	Intervertebral foramina	▶ ARTICULATIONS	Costotransverse
Spinous process			

LUMBAR SPINE: AP, Oblique, Lateral, Lateral Lumbosacral Junction

▶ LUMBAR VERTEBRAE	Transverse process	Intervertebral foramina	Intervertebral disk space
L1–5	Pars interarticularis	▶ T–12	Zygapophyseal joint
Pedicle	Superior articular process	▶ SACRUM	Lumbosacral junction
Spinous process	Inferior articular process	▶ ARTICULATIONS	Sacroiliac

SACRUM: AP, Lateral

▶ SACRUM	Sacral promontory	▶ COCCYX	Lumbosacral
Ala	▶ PELVIS	▶ L–5	Symphysis pubis
Sacral foramina	Ilium	▶ ARTICULATIONS	
Base	Pubis	Sacroiliac	

COCCYX: AP, Lateral

▶ SACRUM	▶ COCCYX	▶ PELVIS	Obturator foramen
	Base	Pubis	Symphysis pubis
	Apex		

COMPLETE THE APPROPRIATE INFORMATION SHEET FOR
EACH DRAWING.

10

VERTEBRAL
COLUMN

► AP CERVICAL SPINE

CENTERING LANDMARK AND CR ORIENTATION

PATIENT POSITIONING

MAIN STRUCTURES VISUALIZED

NOTES

AP CERVICAL SPINE

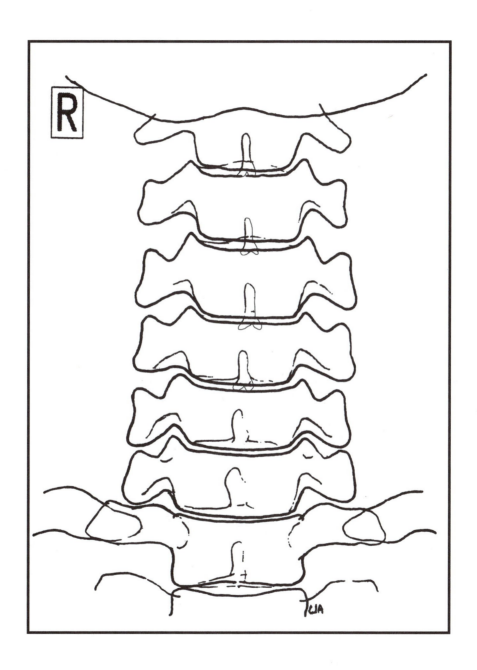

► OBLIQUE CERVICAL SPINE

CENTERING LANDMARK AND CR ORIENTATION

PATIENT POSITIONING

MAIN STRUCTURES VISUALIZED

NOTES

OBLIQUE CERVICAL SPINE

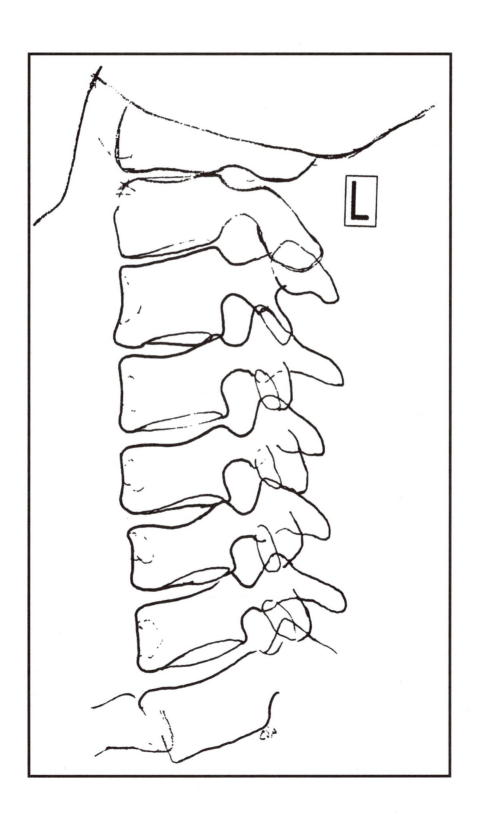

► LATERAL CERVICAL SPINE

CENTERING
LANDMARK AND CR
ORIENTATION

PATIENT
POSITIONING

MAIN STRUCTURES
VISUALIZED

NOTES

LATERAL CERVICAL SPINE

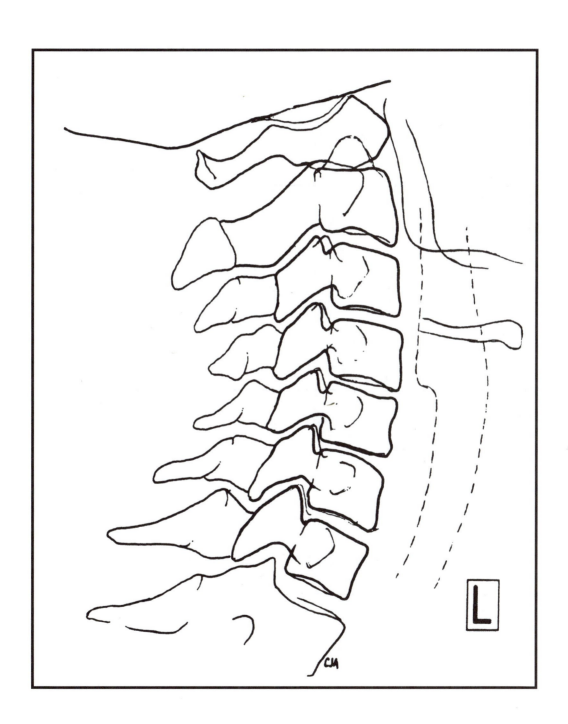

▶ AP ATLAS AND AXIS (OPEN-MOUTH ODONTOID)

CENTERING
LANDMARK AND CR
ORIENTATION

PATIENT
POSITIONING

MAIN STRUCTURES
VISUALIZED

NOTES

AP ATLAS AND AXIS (OPEN-MOUTH ODONTOID)

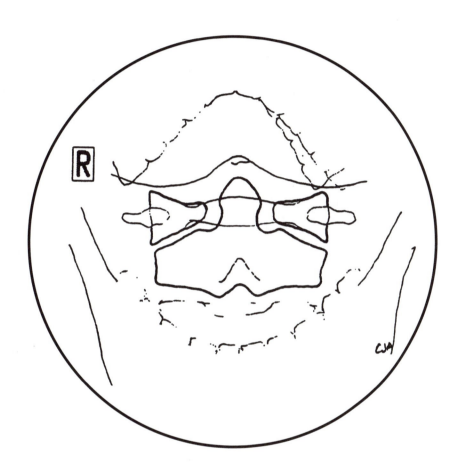

► AP THORACIC SPINE

CENTERING LANDMARK AND CR ORIENTATION

PATIENT POSITIONING

MAIN STRUCTURES VISUALIZED

NOTES

AP THORACIC SPINE

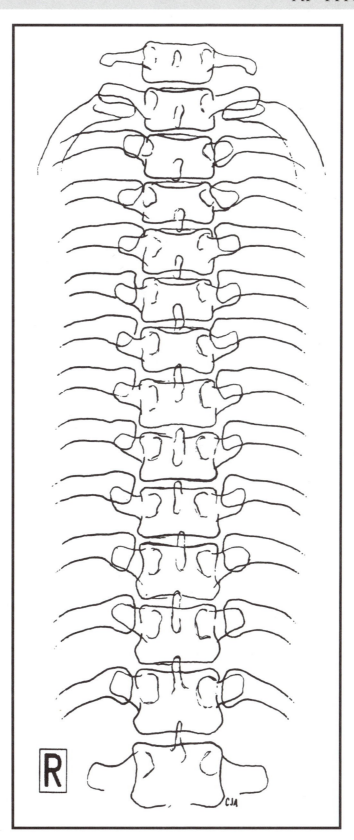

► LATERAL THORACIC SPINE

CENTERING LANDMARK AND CR ORIENTATION

PATIENT POSITIONING

MAIN STRUCTURES VISUALIZED

NOTES

LATERAL THORACIC SPINE

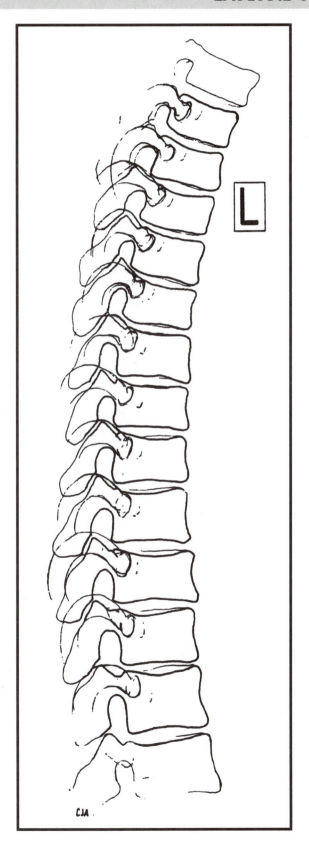

► LATERAL CERVICOTHORACIC REGION (SWIMMER'S)

CENTERING LANDMARK AND CR ORIENTATION

PATIENT POSITIONING

MAIN STRUCTURES VISUALIZED

NOTES

LATERAL CERVICOTHORACIC REGION (SWIMMERS)

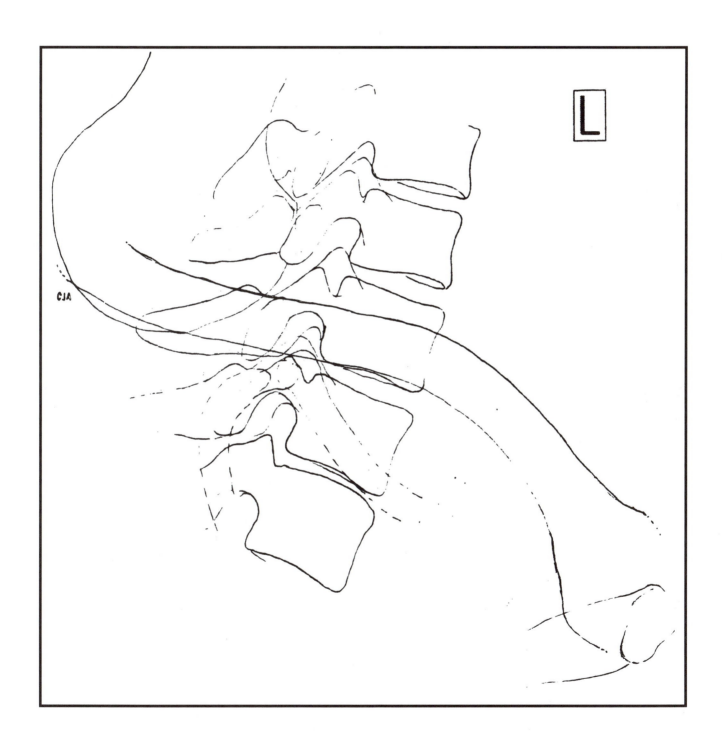

▶ AP LUMBAR SPINE

CENTERING
LANDMARK AND CR
ORIENTATION

PATIENT
POSITIONING

MAIN STRUCTURES
VISUALIZED

NOTES

AP LUMBAR SPINE

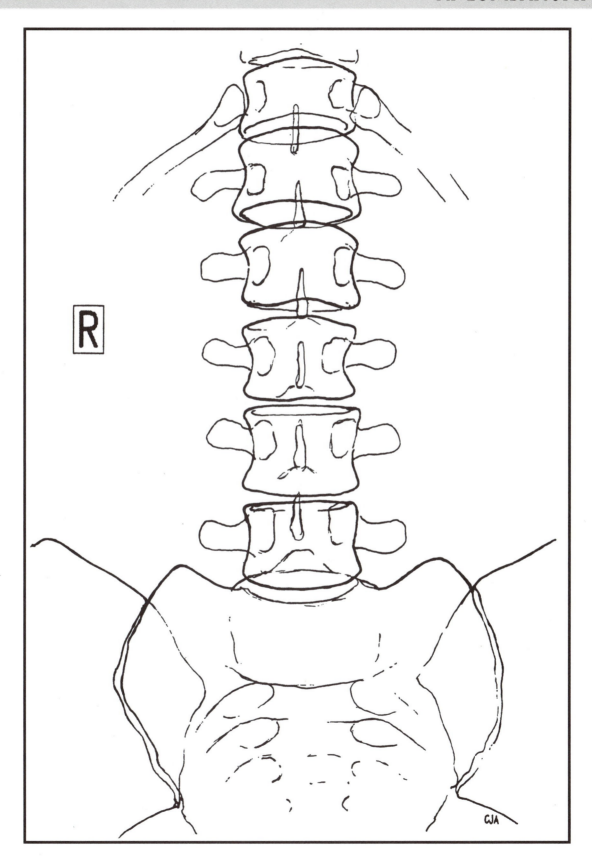

► OBLIQUE LUMBAR SPINE

CENTERING
LANDMARK AND CR
ORIENTATION

PATIENT
POSITIONING

MAIN STRUCTURES
VISUALIZED

NOTES

OBLIQUE LUMBAR SPINE

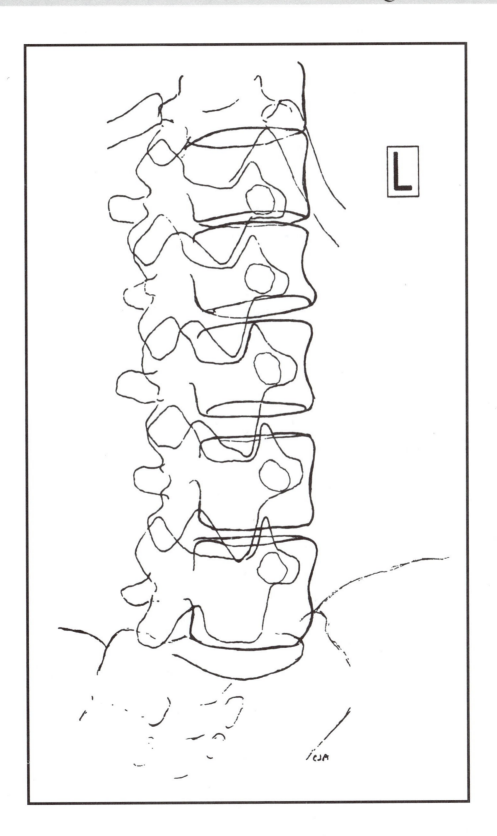

► LATERAL LUMBAR SPINE

CENTERING LANDMARK AND CR ORIENTATION

PATIENT POSITIONING

MAIN STRUCTURES VISUALIZED

NOTES

LATERAL LUMBAR SPINE

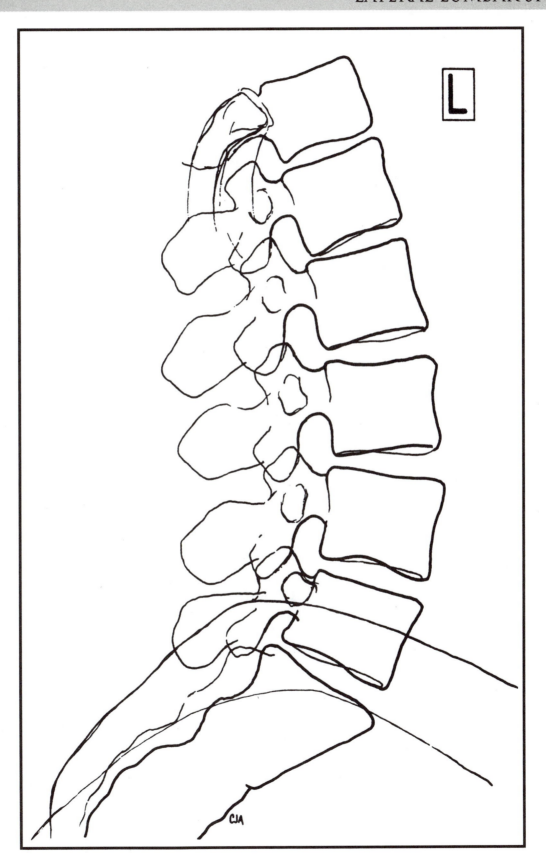

► LATERAL LUMBOSACRAL JUNCTION

CENTERING LANDMARK AND CR ORIENTATION

PATIENT POSITIONING

MAIN STRUCTURES VISUALIZED

NOTES

LATERAL LUMBOSACRAL JUNCTION

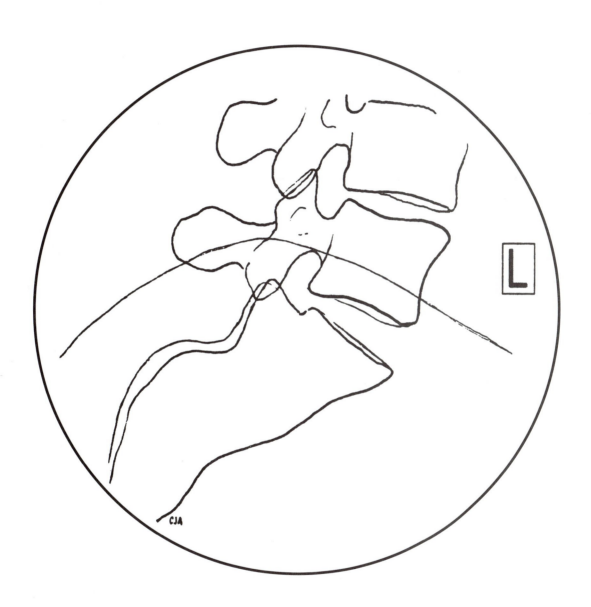

▶ AP SACRUM

CENTERING LANDMARK AND CR ORIENTATION

PATIENT POSITIONING

MAIN STRUCTURES VISUALIZED

NOTES

AP SACRUM

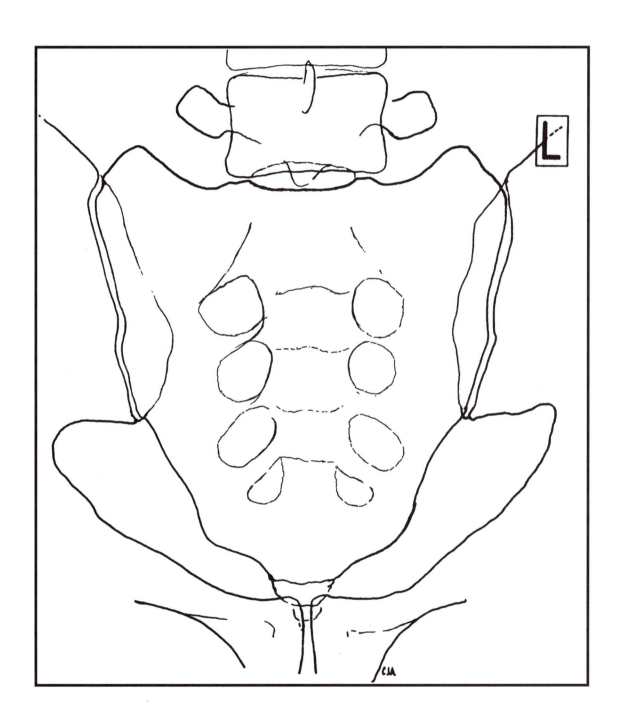

► LATERAL SACRUM

CENTERING LANDMARK AND CR ORIENTATION

PATIENT POSITIONING

MAIN STRUCTURES VISUALIZED

NOTES

LATERAL SACRUM

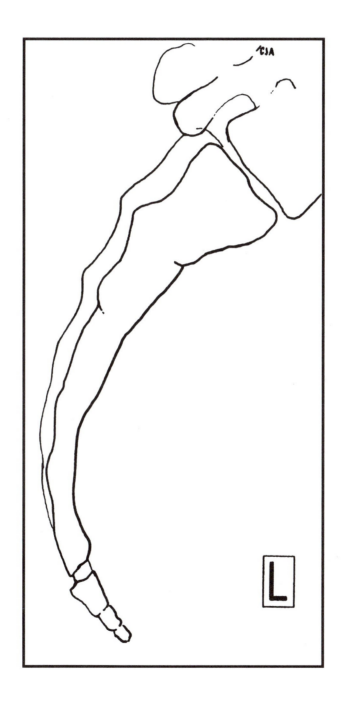

► AP COCCYX

CENTERING LANDMARK AND CR ORIENTATION

PATIENT POSITIONING

MAIN STRUCTURES VISUALIZED

NOTES

AP COCCYX

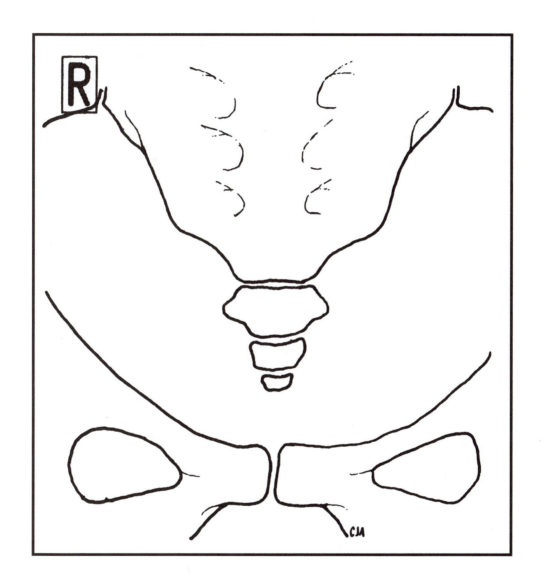

▶ LATERAL COCCYX

CENTERING LANDMARK AND CR ORIENTATION

PATIENT POSITIONING

MAIN STRUCTURES VISUALIZED

NOTES

LATERAL COCCYX

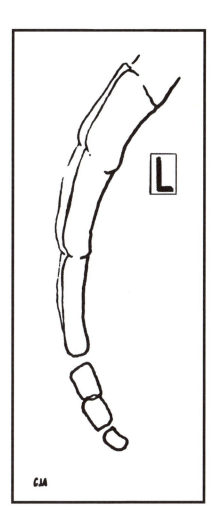

▶ STUDY QUESTIONS

1. Identify the five divisions of the vertebral column:

   _____

   _____

   _____

   _____

   _____

2. There are normally _____ anteroposterior curves in the vertebral column.

3. How does the number of bones in the vertebral column differ between a child and an adult? _____

   _____

4. The _____ and _____ curves are considered to be primary curves because they are present at birth.

5. The _____ and _____ are denoted as secondary curves because they develop when a child holds his head erect and begins to walk.

6. What is a *compensatory curve?* _____

   _____

7. Which curves are described as concave posterior?

   _____

   _____

8. Which curves are described as convex posterior?

   _____

   _____

9. The "hunchback" of Notre Dame has a condition known as _____ , which occurs when the thoracic curvature becomes exaggerated.

10. _____ occurs when the lumbar curve becomes exaggerated and more concave.

11. _____ is an abnormal lateral or S-shaped curvature of the spine.

12. What are the two main parts of a vertebra? _____

   _____

13. The posterior ringlike portion of the vertebra is called the _____ .

14. A vertebra is classified as what type of bone? _____

   _____

15. Which part of the vertebra is considered to be "weight-bearing"? _____

16. The body of the vertebra is primarily formed from _____ (cancellous/compact) bone.

17. Two short stemlike structures called _____ attach the body to the vertebral arch.

18. Through which foramina does the spinal cord pass?

   _____

19. A/an _____ foramen is formed by the inferior vertebral notch of one vertebra and the superior vertebral notch of the vertebra directly below it.

20. On which structure of the vertebra are the superior and inferior vertebral notches located? _____

   _____

21. A broad, flat plate of bone located posteriorly to the pedicle on the vertebral arch is the _____ .

22. List the seven processes that originate from the vertebral arch. _____

   _____

   _____

   _____

   _____

   _____

   _____

23. The pedicles of a cervical vertebra form a _____ ° (degree) angle to the vertebral body.

24. A condition known as _____ occurs when the laminae of a vertebra fail to meet posteriorly at the midline.

25. What forms the *vertebral canal?* _____

   _____

26. The articular processes project upward or downward from the vertebral arch at the junction of the _____ _____ and _____ .

27. The _____ can often be palpated down the midline of a person's back.

28. The bodies of adjacent cervical vertebrae overlap slightly as they slant inferiorly toward their anterior margin at an angle of _____ ° (degrees).

29. The _____ is formed at the point of fusion of the right and left laminae of a vertebra.

30. There are _____ cervical vertebrae, _____ thoracic vertebrae, and _____ lumbar vertebrae.

31. Which cervical vertebra is also known as the "vertebra prominens"? Explain why. _____
_____

32. The _____ processes project laterally from the junction of the pedicles and laminae on a lumbar or thoracic vertebrae.

33. What does the term "bifid" mean and how does it relate to the cervical vertebrae? _____
_____

34. Where is the articular pillar of a cervical vertebra located? (Be specific.) _____
_____

35. List two ways in which the transverse processes of the cervical vertebrae differ from those of the thoracic and lumbar regions. _____
_____

36. Which cervical vertebra is also called the axis? _____

37. Which cervical vertebra is also called the atlas? _____

38. How does C-1 differ structurally from the typical cervical vertebra? _____
_____

39. The articular processes of C-1 are located on the _____ _____ , which is a solid area of bone situated on either side of the vertebral foramen between the anterior and posterior arches.

40. The _____ or _____ is a tooth-shaped process that projects upward from the top of the vertebral body of C-2.

41. Compare the body of a typical thoracic vertebra to the body of a lumbar vertebra. _____
_____

42. The condyles of the occipital bone of the skull articulate with the _____ processes of C-1.

43. Identify the projections that best demonstrate the intervertebral foramina for the following regions of the vertebral column:

cervical _____
thoracic _____
lumbar _____

44. What is a *costal facet;* where is one found in the vertebral column? _____
_____
_____

45. Which region of the vertebral column has spinous processes which are long and slender? _____
_____

46. The _____ is that area on each lamina of a lumbar vertebra between the superior and inferior articular processes.

47. List the structures of a lumbar vertebra that form the parts of the "scotty dog."

nose _____
ear _____
neck _____
eye _____
front leg _____

48. The upper border of the sacrum is the _____ , while the pointed inferior end is the _____ .

49. The sacrum is formed by the fusion of _____ incompletely formed vertebrae.

50. _____ is a condition that occurs when the body of L-5 fuses to the body of the first sacral segment.

51. The four pairs of holes on either surface of the sacrum are known as the _____ _____ .

52. The broad winglike areas of the sacrum, which are situated to either side of the first sacral body, are the _____ _____ .

53. The _____ is the prominent anterior margin of the first sacral segment.

54. Describe the shape and location of the auricular surfaces of the sacrum. _____ _____

55. The opening at the end of the sacral canal on the posterior surface of the sacrum is the _____ _____ .

56. When _____ occurs, the first and second sacral segments have failed to fuse, resulting in a sixth lumbar vertebra.

57. Prior to fusion at the age of 20–30, the sacral segments are separated by _____ .

58. The _____ is a rough ridge of bone running down the midline of the posterior surface of the sacrum.

59. The number of coccygeal segments ranges from _____ to _____ .

60. The _____ are horn-shaped structures projecting upward form the base of the coccyx to articulate with similar structures on the sacrum.

61. The coccyx is usually _____ (less/more) curved on males than on females.

62. The fibrous outer ring of an intervertebral disk is called the _____ .

63. The gelatinous substance comprising the inner portion of an intervertebral disk is the _____ .

64. What is the accurate name for a "slipped disk"? _____ _____

65. Identify the structural and functional (movement) classification of an intervertebral joint. _____ _____

66. What structures are involved in the formation of zygapophyseal joints? _____ _____

67. Identify the projection that will best demonstrate the zygapophyseal joints for the following regions of the vertebral column:
    A. C-1/2   _____
    B. C2–7   _____
    C. Thoracic   _____
    D. Lumbar   _____

68. Describe the location and function of the intervertebral disks. _____ _____ _____

69. Name the joint that permits rotation of the head. _____ _____

70. Name the joint that allows a person to nod her head. ___ _____

71. The _____ joint is formed by the articulation of the head of a rib with the body of a thoracic vertebra.

72. The _____ joint is formed by the articulation of the tubercle of a rib with the transverse process of a thoracic vertebra.

73. What type of movement is permitted by the atlantoaxial joint? _____ _____

74. Match the following vertebrae with their corresponding landmarks.

A. _____ L-4/5   1. symphysis pubis
B. _____ T-10   2. thyroid cartilage
                        3. ASIS
C. _____ Coccyx   4. iliac crest
D. _____ T-2/3   5. xiphoid process
                        6. sternal angle
E. _____ C-4   7. jugular notch
F. _____ L-2/3   8. lower costal margin

75. Why should collars or other immobilization devices be left in place for radiography of the cervical spine unless the radiographer is told by the physician to remove them? _____

76. What SID is used when taking a lateral projection of the cervical spine in an upright position? _____

77. How is the anode-heel effect used effectively for AP and lateral projections of the thoracic spine? _____
_____
_____

78. Why is the use of radiolucent supports under the waist recommended for lateral projections of the thoracic and lumbar vertebrae? _____
_____

79. A hyperflexion/hyperextension study of the cervical spine is performed with the patient erect in a/an _____ _____ position.

80. Why is the PA projection preferred over the AP projection when performing a scoliosis series? _____
_____

81. What is the purpose of using a "breathing technique" for a lateral projection of the thoracic spine? _____
_____

82. What breathing instructions are given for a lateral projection of the lumbar spine to demonstrate as many vertebrae as possible free of superimposition by the diaphragm?_____ .

83. On an AP projection of the cervical spine, the central ray should be directed _____ (degree and direction) to the level of _____ .

84. The patient should be rotated _____° (degrees) for oblique projections of the cervical spine.

85. On an AP projection of the thoracic spine, the central ray is directed perpendicular to the level of _____ .

86. You are viewing a lateral projection of the thoracic spine. How can you determine if rotation is present on the radiograph? _____
_____
_____

87. For a PA oblique projection of the thoracic spine, the patient should be rotated approximately _____° (degrees) from the PA position or _____° (degrees) from the lateral position.

88. Why is it recommended that the patient flex his hips and knees for an AP projection of the lumbar spine? _____
_____

89. An AP oblique projection of the lumbar spine requires that the patient be rotated _____° (degrees) from an AP position.

90. The centering point for an AP projection of the lumbar spine when using a 14 × 17-in. cassette is _____
_____ .

91. To assure that the vertebral column is positioned down the middle of the film on an RPO or LPO of the lumbar spine, the plane passing _____ _____ should be centered to the midline of the table.

92. Which projection(s) of the lumbar spine would be performed to evaluate motion at the site of a spinal fusion?
_____
_____

93. On an AP axial projection of the lumbosacral junction on a female patient, the central ray should be directed _____ (degree and direction) to the level of _____ .

94. What is the purpose of placing lead masking on the table behind the patient for lateral projections of the vertebral column? _____

_____

_____

95. The centering point for a lateral projection of the lumbosacral junction is _____ .

96. Indicate the degree and direction of the central ray for AP projections of the following structures:

    A. sacrum _____

    B. coccyx _____

97. Which projection of the sacrum will best demonstrate the sacral promontory? _____

98. The centering point for an AP projection of the coccyx is

_____ .

99. For each of the items below, identify the projection that best demonstrates the anatomy:

    A. right intervertebral foramina of the cervical spine

    _____

    B. superimposed pedicles of the lumbar spine

    _____

    C. spinous processes of the thoracic spine in profile

    _____

    D. left pedicles of the cervical vertebrae

    _____

    E. right zygapophyseal joint between L-2/3

    _____

    F. right zygapophyseal joint between T-6/7

    _____

    G. superimposition of the anterior and posterior sacral foramina

    _____

    H. subluxation of L-2

    _____

    I. superimposed articular pillars of C-4

    _____

    J. abnormal lateral curvature of scoliosis

    _____

100. Complete the following table:

Projection	CR Angle/Angle of Part	Centering Point	Film Size	Structures Seen
RPO cervical spine				
LPO thoracic spine				
Lateral cervicothoracic region				
LPO lumbar spine				
Lateral coccyx				

► CASE STUDIES

1. A 65-year-old male is sent to the radiology department for radiographs of the lumbar spine. He is experiencing pain in the right sciatic region and has a possible diagnosis of spondylolisthesis or a herniated disk. When the patient is positioned in the lateral position, you notice that his chest is very broad and his spine is not parallel to the table.

   ► Explain how you would compensate for the hypersthenic build of this patient on the lateral and L5–S1 spot projections of the lumbar spine.

   ► Describe how spondylolisthesis would look on the radiographs.

   ► What part of the disk actually herniates? How would this appear radiographically? What alternate radiographic procedure would better visualize this pathology?

2. An unexpected ice storm has brought an influx of injured patients to the emergency department. Your next patient is a 52-year-old female who slipped down her icy steps and landed on her tailbone. She is lying prone on a stretcher and tells you that she couldn't possibly lie on her back. Radiographic examination of the sacrum and coccyx has been ordered.

   ► How must you modify the examination due to the patient's position?

   ► Discuss how this modification will affect centering and central ray orientation.

3. After falling 15 ft from a balcony, a patient is brought into the emergency room with a possible thoracic spine injury. Even though her cervical spine has been cleared, she is unable to roll on her side for the lateral and swimmer's lateral projections.

   ► Discuss the method you will use to obtain the three routine projections of the thoracic spine.

4. An 82-year-old female has been sent to the imaging department by her physician for radiographs of her thoracic spine. She is extremely kyphotic and appears very frail. She states that she has been experiencing pain in her upper back for some time with no known injury. She is unable to lie on her back.

  ▸ How does the patient's appearance relate to the technical factors used for the radiographs?

  ▸ Discuss the method you will use to obtain the three routine projections of the thoracic spine.

  ▸ The completed radiographic examination revealed a compression fracture of T-5. How could this occur without any traumatic injury?

  ....

  ....

  ....

  ....

  ....

  ....

  ....

  ....

  ....

5. Your patient has sustained a serious neck injury in a motor vehicle accident. She has been brought to trauma x-ray on a backboard with a cervical collar on her neck. The cervical spine series that has been requested includes AP, lateral, open-mouth odontoid, and both oblique projections. You have taken the lateral cervical spine radiograph and the neck has *not* been cleared because C-7 was not adequately visualized.

  ▸ Explain how you will proceed with the rest of the series without removing the collar.

  ▸ What can you do to better demonstrate C-7?

  ....

  ....

  ....

  ....

  ....

  ....

  ....

  ....

▶ POSITIONING WORKSHEETS

COLOR THE FOLLOWING ANATOMICAL PARTS ON THE DRAW-
INGS FOR THIS SECTION. LABEL ALL PARTS THAT CAN BE SEEN
ON EACH POSITION OR PROJECTION. LABEL THE ANGLE OF
THE CR AND THE DEGREE OF HEAD ROTATION ON THE SMALL
HEAD DRAWINGS WHERE APPROPRIATE.

SKULL: PA (0°), PA (15° Caldwell), Lateral, AP Axial (Towne)

▶ FRONTAL BONE	▶ PARIETAL BONE	Frontal	▶ MANDIBLE
▶ TEMPORAL BONE	▶ OCCIPITAL BONE	Maxillary	▶ DENS
Petrous pyramid	▶ ORBITS	Ethmoid	▶ BONY NASAL SEPTUM
Mastoid air cells	▶ FORAMEN MAGNUM	Sphenoid	
Mastoid process	▶ SINUSES	▶ MAXILLA	

MASTOIDS: Mod. Lateral (Law), Posterior Profile (Stenvers), Axiolateral (Schuller), Axiolateral Oblique (Mayer)

▶ TEMPORAL BONE	Mastoid process	▶ INTERNAL ACOUSTIC	▶ DENS
Mastoid air cells	▶ EAM	(AUDITORY) CANAL	

COMPLETE THE APPROPRIATE INFORMATION SHEET FOR
EACH DRAWING.

11

SKULL

▶ PA SKULL (0°)

CENTERING LANDMARK AND CR ORIENTATION

PATIENT POSITIONING

MAIN STRUCTURES VISUALIZED

NOTES

PA SKULL (0°)

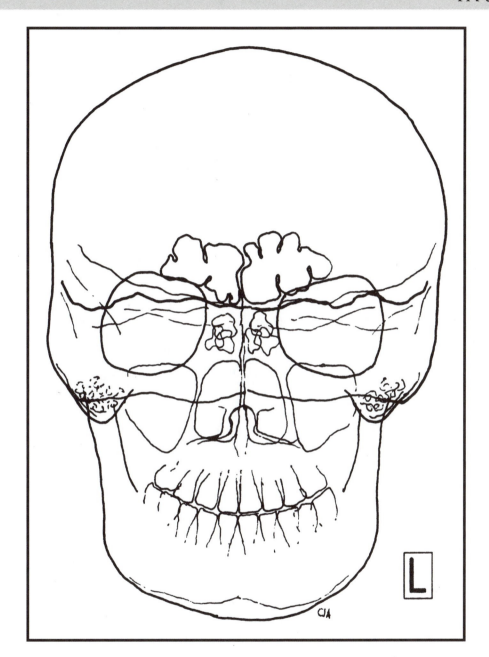

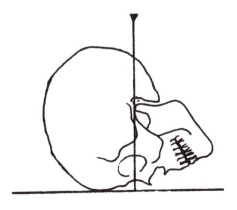

► PA SKULL (15° CALDWELL)

CENTERING LANDMARK AND CR ORIENTATION

PATIENT POSITIONING

MAIN STRUCTURES VISUALIZED

NOTES

PA SKULL (15° CALDWELL)

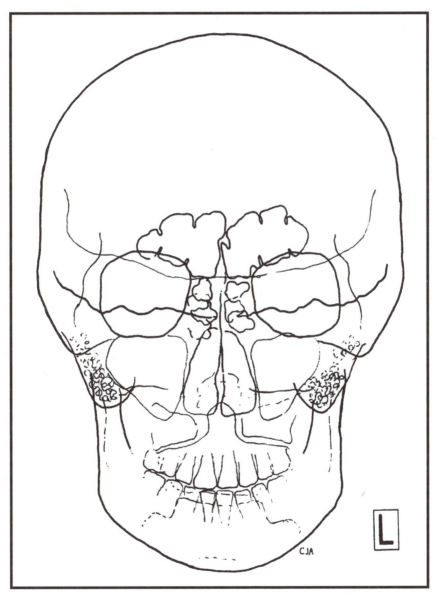

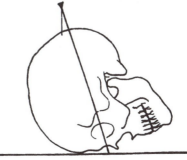

► LATERAL SKULL

CENTERING LANDMARK AND CR ORIENTATION

PATIENT POSITIONING

MAIN STRUCTURES VISUALIZED

NOTES

LATERAL SKULL

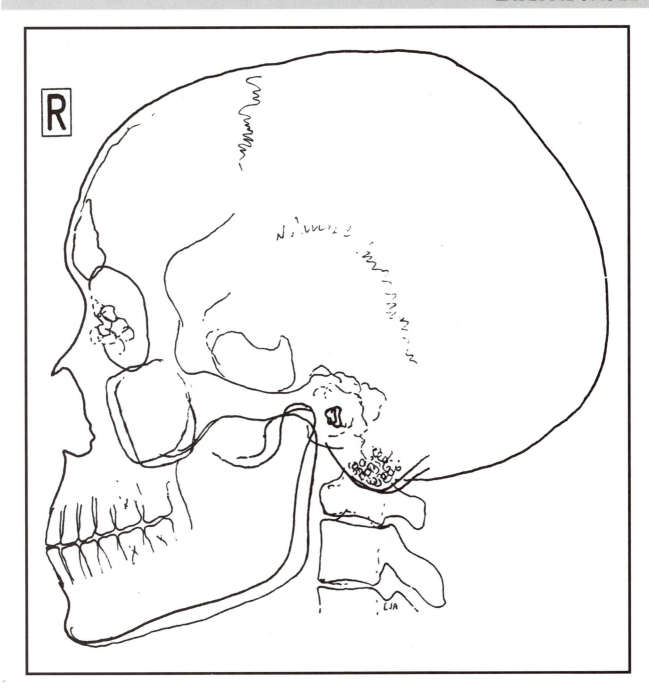

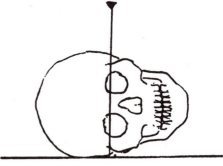

► AP AXIAL SKULL (TOWNE)

CENTERING LANDMARK AND CR ORIENTATION

PATIENT POSITIONING

MAIN STRUCTURES VISUALIZED

NOTES

AP AXIAL SKULL (TOWNE)

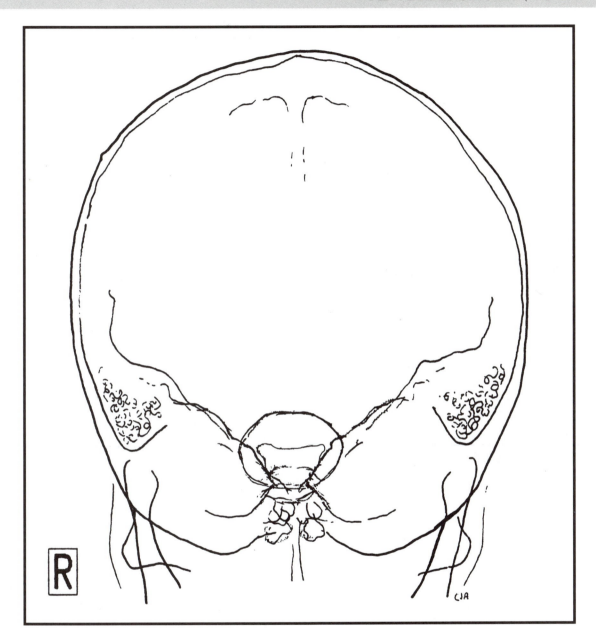

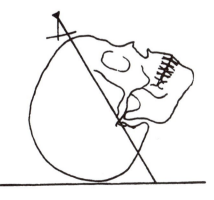

► MODIFIED LATERAL (LAW) MASTOIDS

CENTERING LANDMARK AND CR ORIENTATION

PATIENT POSITIONING

MAIN STRUCTURES VISUALIZED

NOTES

MODIFIED LATERAL (LAW) MASTOIDS

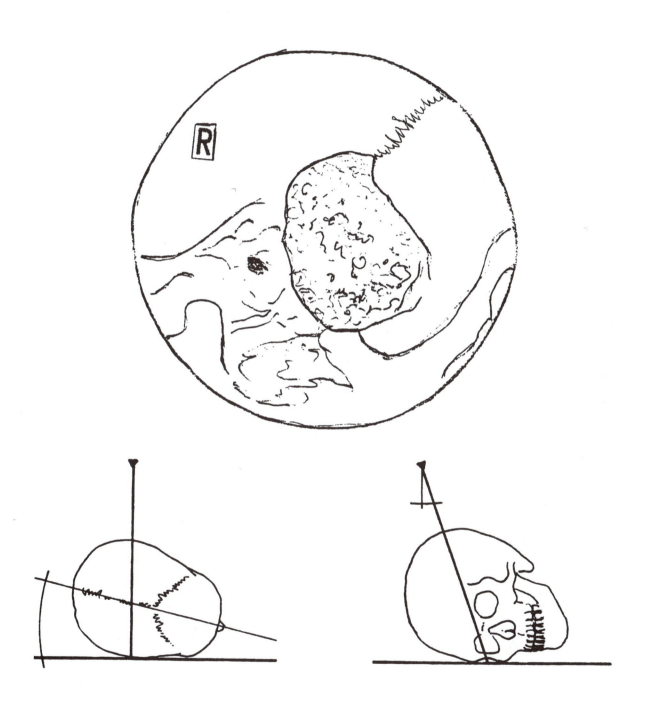

▶ POSTERIOR PROFILE (STENVERS) MASTOIDS

CENTERING LANDMARK AND CR ORIENTATION

PATIENT POSITIONING

MAIN STRUCTURES VISUALIZED

NOTES

POSTERIOR PROFILE (STENVERS) MASTOIDS

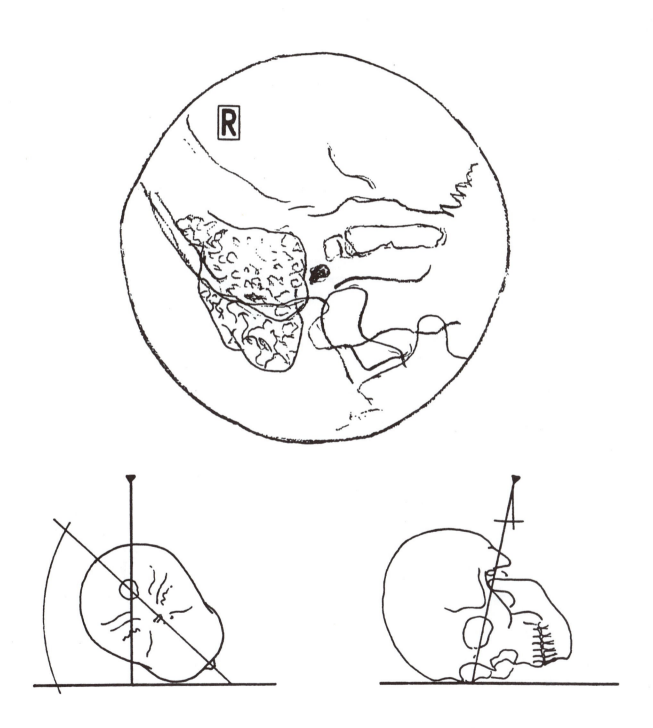

► AXIOLATERAL (SCHULLER) MASTOIDS

CENTERING LANDMARK AND CR ORIENTATION

PATIENT POSITIONING

MAIN STRUCTURES VISUALIZED

NOTES

AXIOLATERAL (SCHULLER) MASTOIDS

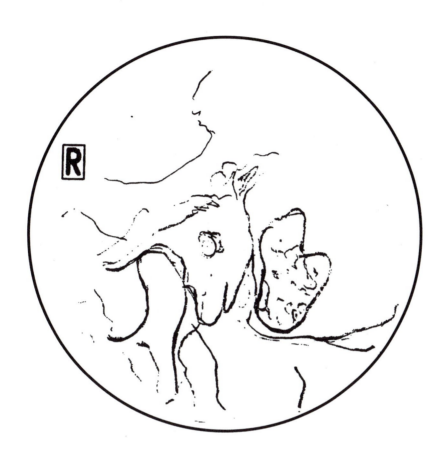

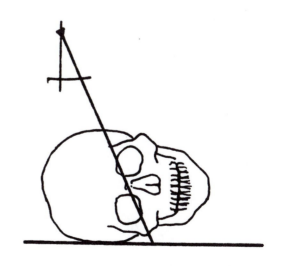

▶ AXIOLATERAL OBLIQUE (MAYER) MASTOIDS

CENTERING
LANDMARK AND CR
ORIENTATION

PATIENT
POSITIONING

MAIN STRUCTURES
VISUALIZED

NOTES

AXIOLATERAL OBLIQUE (MAYER) MASTOIDS

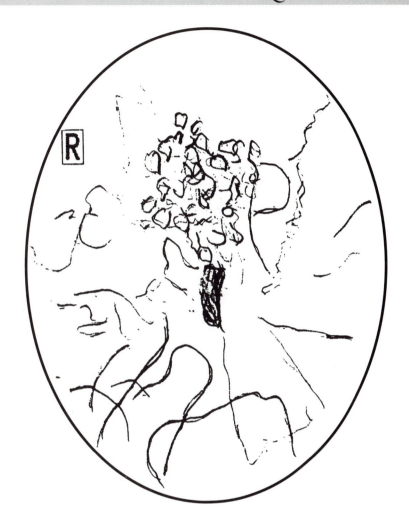

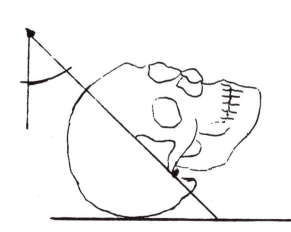

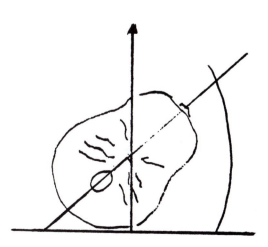

► STUDY QUESTIONS

1. What is the cranial vault? _____

_____

2. List the bones of the calvarium and the cranial floor.

_____
_____
_____
_____
_____
_____
_____

3. The skull is divided into _____ cranial bones and _____ facial bones.

4. The four bones forming the skull cap are classified as _____ type of bones, while the four bones forming the cranial floor are classified as _____ type of bones.

5. The inner and outer tables of the bones of the calvarium are formed from _____ bone, and the middle layer between them is formed from _____ bone.

6. What is *diploe?* _____
_____
_____

7. The two main parts of the frontal bone are the _____ portion and the _____ portion.

8. Which of the bones of the calvarium are square and articulate with each other at the sagittal suture? _____

9. The _____ bone forms the posteroinferior portion of the calvarium.

10. The _____ bone is located between the orbits to form the medial walls of the orbits and lateral walls of the nasal cavity.

11. Which of the cranial bones acts as an anchor or keystone to hold the eight cranial bones together? _____ _____

12. Which cranial bone is involved in the formation of the zygomatic arch? _____

13. The _____ portion of the frontal bone forms the forehead.

14. The curved ridges of bone located beneath the eyebrows on the frontal bone are called the _____ _____ .

15. Describe the location of the frontal sinuses on the frontal bone. _____
_____

16. The _____ of the frontal bone form the roof of the orbits and part of the floor of the cranial fossa.

17. The orbital portion of the frontal bone articulates posteriorly with the _____ bone.

18. An arched or horseshoe-shaped opening between the orbital plates of the frontal bone is known as the _____ .

19. The two _____ bones form the roof and lateral walls of the cranium.

20. Small palpable bumps located on either side of the upper forehead are called the _____ .

21. The widest point of the skull can be measured between the _____ .

22. The spinal cord passes through a large hole in the occipital bone known as the _____ .

23. What is the name of the palpable bump located on the midline of the back of the head? _____

24. Where is the clivus located? _____
_____

25. The _____ lines are two parallel ridges that run horizontally on the occipital bone and serve as the attachment site for muscles.

26. The occipital condyles articulate with the first cervical vertebra to form the _____ joint.

27. The cribiform plate forms the _____ portion of the ethmoid bone and articulates with the _____ of the frontal bone.

28. What is the function of the numerous perforations in the cribiform plate? _____ _____

29. A triangular bony process projecting upward from the cribiform plate is known as the _____ _____ or rooster's comb.

30. The ethmoid sinuses are contained in thin, spongelike structures called _____ or _____ .

31. The superior and middle nasal conchae are also known as _____ .

32. Specifically, which part(s) of the ethmoid bone form(s) the medial orbital walls and lateral walls of the nasal cavity? _____

33. What function do the nasal conchae perform? _____ _____

34. The hollow central portion of the sphenoid bone is the _____ .

35. The sella turcica is bordered anteriorly by the _____ _____ and posteriorly by the _____ _____ .

36. Specifically, which part(s) of the sphenoid bone articulate(s) with the frontal bone? _____ _____

37. The saddle-shaped depression located on the superior aspect of the body of the sphenoid bone is called the _____ .

38. The foramina rotundum, ovale, spinosum, and lacerum are located on the _____ of the sphenoid bone.

39. The _____ are bony extensions that project inferiorly from the sphenoid bone.

40. A split or cleft between the greater and lesser wings of the sphenoid bone is known as the _____ _____ .

41. The _____ is an important structure of the endocrine system that is housed in the sella turcica.

42. Identify the four regions of the temporal bone. _____ , _____ _____ , _____

43. The thin _____ portion of the temporal bone forms part of the cranial wall above the ear.

44. The _____ is a slender spike of bone projecting inferiorly from the tympanic portion of the temporal bone.

45. The rounded bump on the temporal bone, which can be palpated just behind a person's ear, is the _____ _____ .

46. The densest part of the temporal bone is the _____ _____ portion, while the thinnest part is the _____ portion.

47. The petrous ridges lie at a _____ ° (degree) angle to the midsagittal plane in a mesocephalic head.

48. The cartilaginous structure of the ear, which directs sound waves into the external acoustic canal, is the _____ or _____ .

49. The middle ear is an air-filled chamber that is also known as the _____ .

50. A thin, semitransparent structure called the _____ _____ forms the eardrum.

51. Name the auditory ossicles: _____ , _____ , _____

52. On your last airplane flight, your felt a "popping" sensation in your ears. Why did this occur and what structures were involved? _____ _____ _____

53. Identify the five communications of the middle ear.

_____

_____

_____

_____

_____

54. The two basic divisions of the inner ear are the _____ _____ and the _____ _____ .

55. The spiral-shaped _____ of the inner ear houses the receptors for hearing.

56. The organ(s) of equilibrium is/are the _____ _____ .

57. When referring to the internal ear, what is meant by the phrase "a closed system"? _____

_____

_____

58. Define *suture*. _____

_____

59. The _____ suture is located between the frontal and both parietal bones.

60. The two parietal bones articulate with each other at the _____ suture.

61. The _____ suture is formed between the parietal bones and the occipital bone on the back of the head.

62. The _____ suture is located on the side of the head between the temporal and parietal bones.

63. Structurally, sutures are _____ joints, which are classified according to function as _____ _____ .

64. A/an _____ is a "soft spot" on a neonate's skull.

65. What is a wormian bone? _____

_____

66. On an adult skull, the point of articulation between the frontal and both parietal bones at the anterior end of the sagittal suture is known as the _____ .

67. On an adult skull, the point of articulation between the occipital bone and both parietal bones at the posterior end of the sagittal suture is known as the _____ _____ .

68. On an infant's skull, the _____ fontanel is located between the frontal and both parietal bones.

69. The posterolateral fontanel is also called the _____ _____ fontanel on an infant's skull and the _____ on an adult's skull.

70. Name the bones that articulate at the anterolateral fontanel on an infant's skull. _____

_____

FOR QUESTIONS 71–85, MATCH THE FOLLOW-ING STRUCTURES WITH THE BONE ON WHICH THEY ARE LOCATED.

F = FRONTAL   P = PARIETAL
T = TEMPORAL   O = OCCIPITAL
E = ETHMOID   S = SPHENOID

71. _____ inion

72. _____ crista galli

73. _____ petrous ridges

74. _____ mandibular fossa

75. _____ pterygoid processes

76. _____ lateral masses or labyrinths

77. _____ orbital plates

78. _____ zygomatic process

79. _____ superior and middle nasal conchae

80. _____ foramen magnum

81. _____ dorsum sellae

82. _____ clinoid processes

83. _____ ethmoidal notch

84. _____ superior nuchal lines

85. _____ mastoid air cells

86. _____ is a term that describes a long, narrow, and deep head.

87. The landmark located on the midline at the junction of the upper lip and nose is the _____ .

88. The inner and outer _____ are located at the junctions of the upper and lower eyelids.

89. The _____ is the topographical landmark located at the slight depression at the bridge of the nose, which corresponds with the frontonasal suture.

90. The supraorbital margin is located on the _____ _____ bone.

91. The smooth, triangular area located above the bridge of the nose and between the eyebrows is the _____ _____ .

92. A positioning line extending from the outer canthus of the eye to the EAM is the _____ .

93. The _____ divides the head into equal right and left halves.

94. There is approximately _____ ° (degrees) difference between the orbitomeatal and infraorbitomeatal lines.

95. On an AP axial projection of the skull, the central ray should be directed _____ (degree and direction) when the IOML is perpendicular to the film plane.

96. The most superior point on the head is the _____ _____ .

97. Describe the location of the dorsum sellae on an AP axial projection of the skull. _____ _____

98. The petrous ridges are demonstrated in the lower third of the orbits when a _____ (degree and direction) angle is used on a PA (Caldwell) projection of the skull.

99. You are viewing an AP projection of the skull taken on a trauma patient. How can rotation be determined on the radiograph? _____ _____

100. On a lateral projection of the skull, the radiographer should direct the central ray perpendicular to a point _____ .

101. Describe the effect tilt has on a lateral projection of the skull. _____ _____

102. Describe the relationship (parallel or perpendicular) of the following lines and plane to the film plane on a lateral projection of the skull:
    ▸ IOML _____
    ▸ midsagittal plane _____
    ▸ interpupillary line _____

103. Which projection of the skull will demonstrate the following structures: right and left petrous portions at a 47° angle to the midsagittal plane, the foramen magnum, the sphenoid sinuses, and the arch-shaped mandible? _____

104. Which projection of the petrous portions demonstrates the internal and external acoustic meati superimposed? _____

105. The _____ projection demonstrates the petrous portion of the temporal bone along its long axis.

106. Which projection of the skull will demonstrate the superimposed parietal bones? _____ _____

107. What is the centering point for a submentovertical projection of the skull? _____ _____

108. The central ray should be perpendicular to the _____ _____ line on a submentovertical projection of the skull.

109. Why is it recommended that a patient suspend respiration for radiography of the skull? _____
_____

110. The modified lateral (Law method) projection for petrous portions requires that the patient's midsagittal plane be rotated _____ ° (degrees) from a true lateral position and the central ray be directed _____ (degree and direction) to the film.

111. On an axiolateral oblique (Mayer method) projection for petrous portions, the patient's midsagittal plane is rotated at a _____ ° (degrees) angle to the film plane and the central ray is directed _____ (degree and direction).

112. Your patient's forehead, nose, and right cheek are positioned on the table, the midsagittal plane is rotated 45°, and the central ray is directed approximately 12° cephalad. Identify this projection and the anatomy best demonstrated. _____
_____
_____

113. In what direction should the radiographer direct the central ray so that it is perpendicular to the IOML on a verticosubmental projection of the skull? _____
_____

114. Complete the following table:

Projection	CR Angle/Angle of Part	Centering Point	Film Size	Structures Seen
PA skull				
Right axiolateral oblique (Mayer)				
Anterior profile (Arcelin)				
Collimated lateral for sella turcica				
AP axial (Towne)				

▶ CASE STUDIES

1. A 2-year-old child fell, striking his head against a concrete step. He was brought to the emergency department by his mother, where a physician ordered a skull series. The child sustained a 2-in. wound in the middle of his forehead, which required suturing before the radiographs could be taken. As you bring him into the radiographic room, his mother tells you that the child is very upset due to the suturing and will probably kick and scream during the procedure.

   ▶ What skull projections will you take?

   ▶ Since the child is uncooperative, how will you take the radiographs without motion?

   ▶ Discuss the procedure and patient care skills needed in this case.

2. An elderly female patient has been transported to the radiology department by stretcher for radiographic examination of the mastoids. Because the patient is extremely kyphotic, her head is elevated on several pillows. She tells you that she could not have a CT scan of this area because she could not lie on her back long enough to complete the study. The routine series for mastoids at your clinical site includes AP axial (Towne), both axiolateral obliques (Mayer), SMV, and both modified laterals (Law).

▶ Discuss any modifications you may have to make to the procedure in order to complete the radiographic examination on this patient.

▶ Describe the precautions you will take in moving and positioning this patient.

COLOR THE FOLLOWING ANATOMIC PARTS ON THE DRAW-
INGS FOR THIS SECTION. LABEL ALL PARTS THAT CAN BE SEEN
ON EACH POSITION OR PROJECTION. LABEL THE ANGLE OF
THE CR AND THE DEGREE OF HEAD ROTATION ON THE SMALL
HEAD DRAWINGS WHERE APPROPRIATE.

SINUSES: Parietoacanthial (Waters), Lateral, PA (Caldwell), SMV

- ► SINUSES
- Frontal
- Maxillary
- Ethmoid
- Sphenoid
- ► ORBITS
- ► DENS
- ► FRONTAL BONE
- ► TEMPORAL BONE
- Petrous pyramid
- ► MAXILLA
- ► BONY NASAL SEPTUM
- ► SELLA TURCICA

FACIAL BONES: General: Parietoacanthial (Waters), Lateral, Parietoacanthial Modification
Mandible: AP Axial (Towne), Axiolateral Oblique, PA
Zygoma: SMV. Tangential
Nasal Bones: Lateral
Optic Foramen: Parieto-orbital Oblique (Rhese)

- ► FRONTAL BONE
- Frontal sinus
- ► TEMPORAL BONE
- Petrous pyramids
- Mastoids
- EAM
- ► MANDIBLE
- Mandibular condyle
- Coronoid process
- Ramus
- Body
- Mandibular angle
  (gonion)
- Alveolar process
- ► ORBITS
- Optic foramen
- ► MAXILLA
- Maxillary sinus
- Anterior nasal spine
- ► DENS
- ► HYOID BONE
- ► NASAL BONE
- ► ZYGOMATIC ARCH
- ► BONY NASAL SEPTUM

COMPLETE THE APPROPRIATE INFORMATION SHEET FOR
EACH DRAWING.

12

FACIAL BONES &
PARANASAL
SINUSES

► LATERAL SINUSES

CENTERING
LANDMARK AND CR
ORIENTATION

PATIENT
POSITIONING

MAIN STRUCTURES
VISUALIZED

► PARIETOACANTHIAL (WATERS) SINUSES

CENTERING
LANDMARK AND CR
ORIENTATION

PATIENT
POSITIONING

MAIN STRUCTURES
VISUALIZED

LATERAL SINUSES

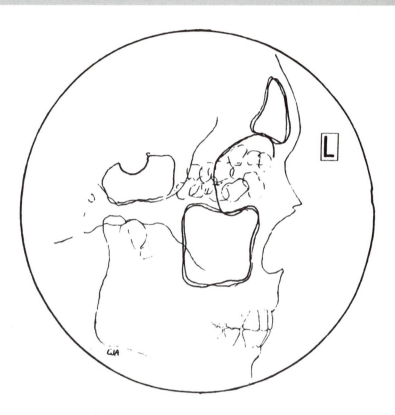

PARIETOACANTHIAL (WATERS) SINUSES

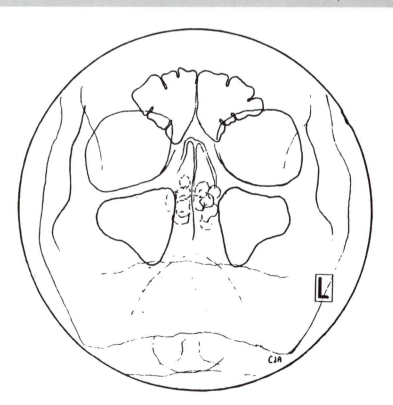

► SUBMENTOVERTICAL SINUSES

CENTERING
LANDMARK AND CR
ORIENTATION

PATIENT
POSITIONING

MAIN STRUCTURES
VISUALIZED

► PA (CALDWELL) SINUSES

CENTERING
LANDMARK AND CR
ORIENTATION

PATIENT
POSITIONING

MAIN STRUCTURES
VISUALIZED

SUBMENTOVERTICAL SINUSES

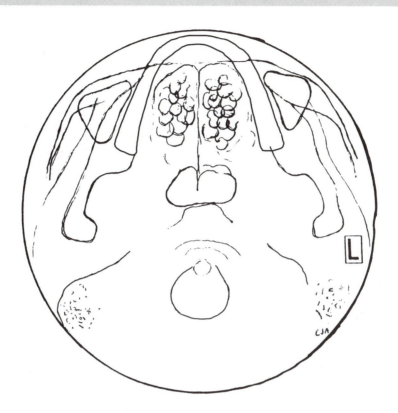

PA (CALDWELL) SINUSES

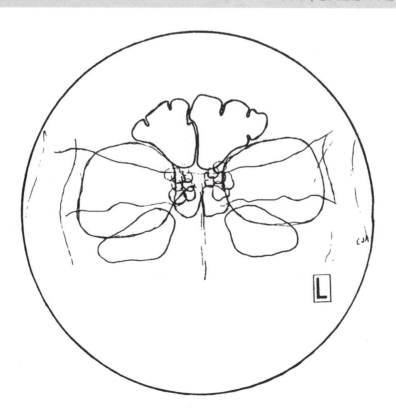

▶ PARIETOACANTHIAL (WATERS) FACIAL BONES

CENTERING
LANDMARK AND CR
ORIENTATION

PATIENT
POSITIONING

MAIN STRUCTURES
VISUALIZED

NOTES

PARIETOACANTHIAL (WATERS) FACIAL BONES

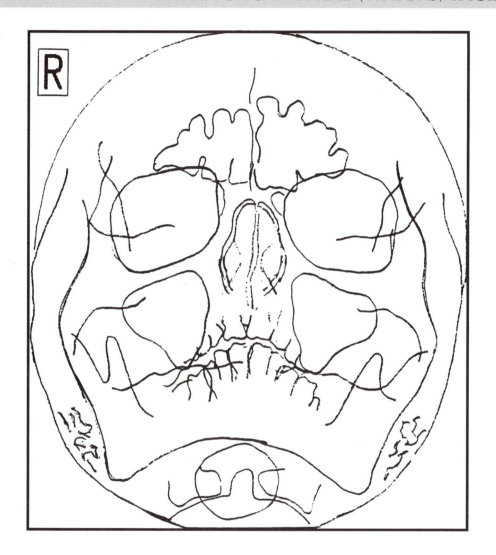

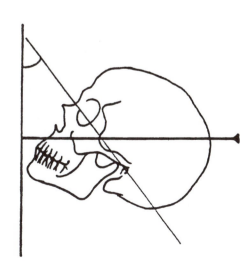

▶ LATERAL FACIAL BONES

CENTERING
LANDMARK AND CR
ORIENTATION

PATIENT
POSITIONING

MAIN STRUCTURES
VISUALIZED

NOTES

LATERAL FACIAL BONES

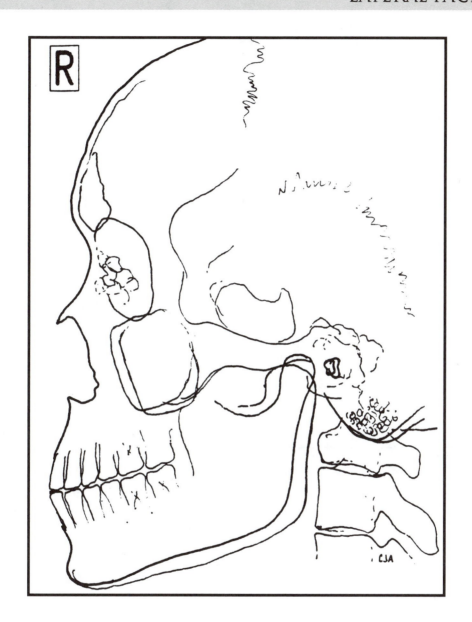

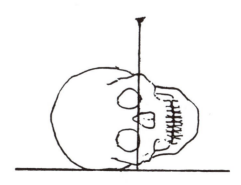

▶ PARIETOACANTHIAL MODIFICATION

CENTERING LANDMARK AND CR ORIENTATION

PATIENT POSITIONING

MAIN STRUCTURES VISUALIZED

NOTES

PARIETOACANTHIAL MODIFICATION

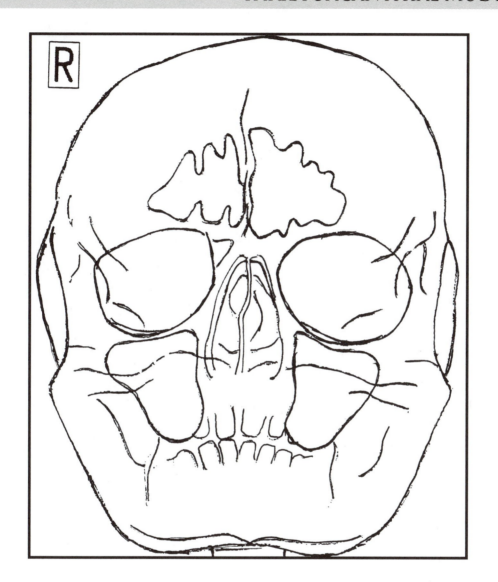

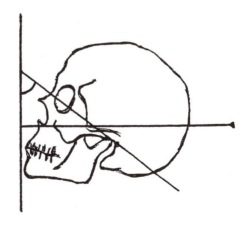

► AP AXIAL (TOWNE) MANDIBLE

CENTERING LANDMARK AND CR ORIENTATION

PATIENT POSITIONING

MAIN STRUCTURES VISUALIZED

NOTES

AP AXIAL (TOWNE) MANDIBLE

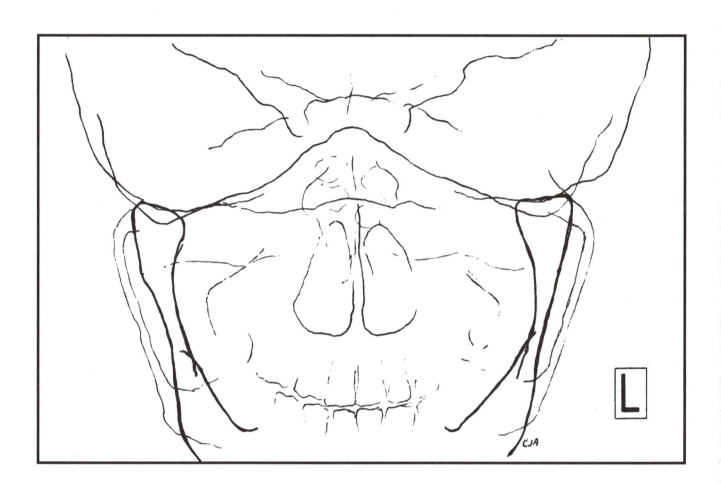

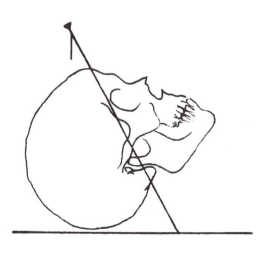

► AXIOLATERAL OBLIQUE MANDIBLE

CENTERING
LANDMARK AND CR
ORIENTATION

PATIENT
POSITIONING

MAIN STRUCTURES
VISUALIZED

NOTES

AXIOLATERAL OBLIQUE MANDIBLE

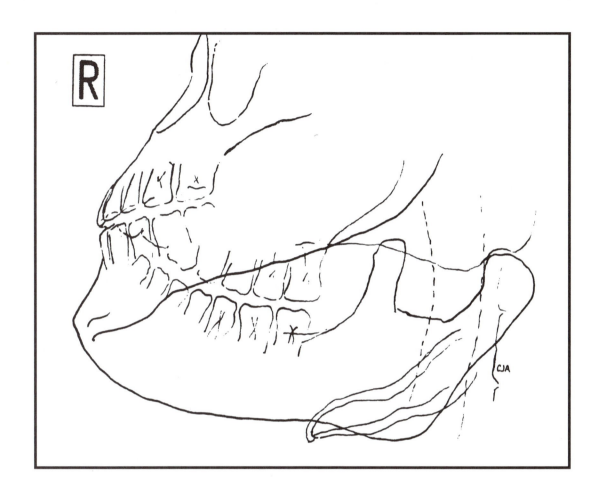

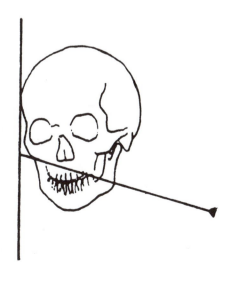

► PA MANDIBLE

CENTERING LANDMARK AND CR ORIENTATION

PATIENT POSITIONING

MAIN STRUCTURES VISUALIZED

NOTES

PA MANDIBLE

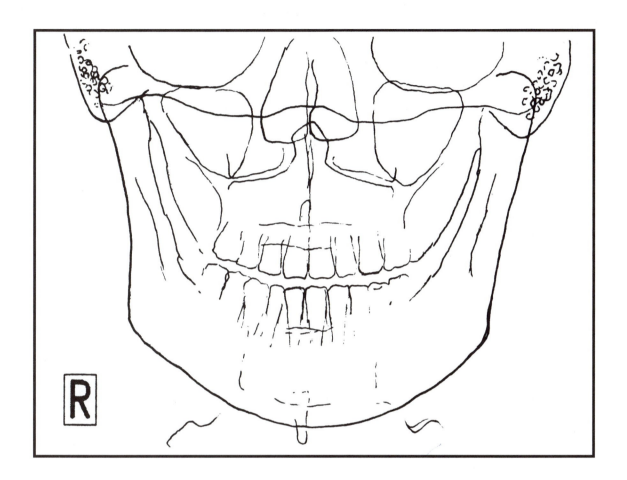

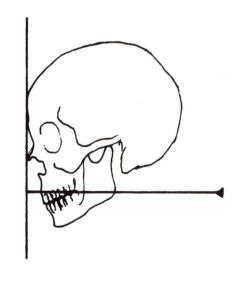

► SUBMENTOVERTICAL ZYGOMA

CENTERING
LANDMARK AND CR
ORIENTATION

PATIENT
POSITIONING

MAIN STRUCTURES
VISUALIZED

► TANGENTIAL ZYGOMA

CENTERING
LANDMARK AND CR
ORIENTATION

PATIENT
POSITIONING

MAIN STRUCTURES
VISUALIZED

SUBMENTOVERTICAL ZYGOMA

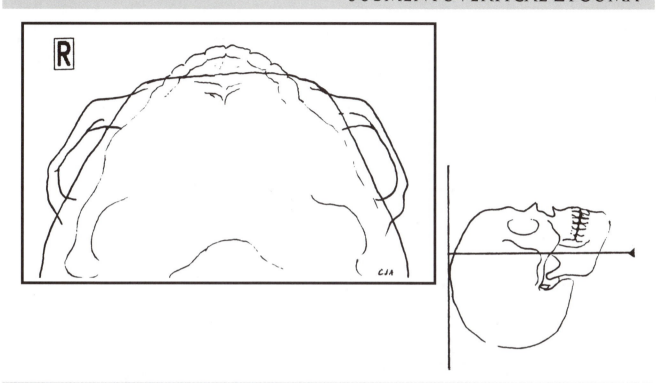

TANGENTIAL ZYGOMA

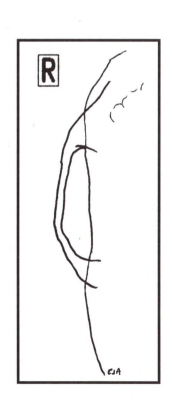

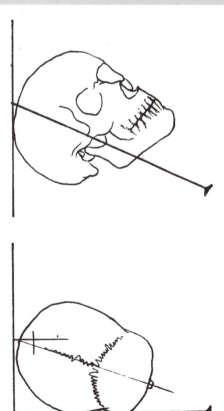

► LATERAL NASAL BONES

**CENTERING
LANDMARK AND CR
ORIENTATION**

**PATIENT
POSITIONING**

**MAIN STRUCTURES
VISUALIZED**

NOTES

LATERAL NASAL BONES

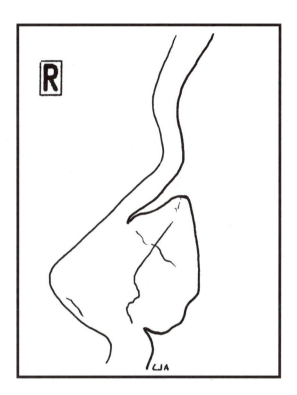

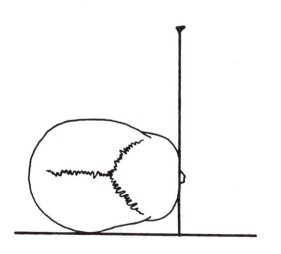

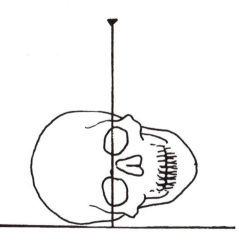

► PARIETO-ORBITAL OBLIQUE (RHESE)

CENTERING LANDMARK AND CR ORIENTATION

PATIENT POSITIONING

MAIN STRUCTURES VISUALIZED

NOTES

PARIETO-ORBITAL OBLIQUE (RHESE)

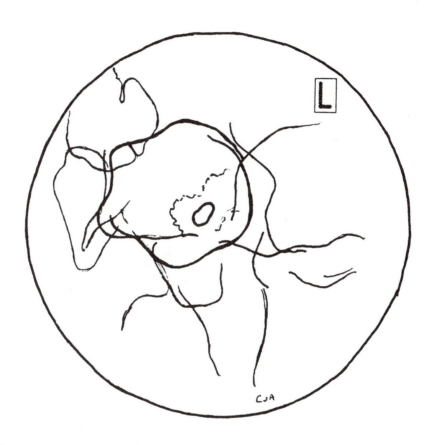

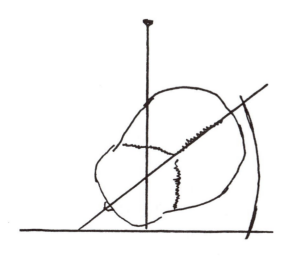

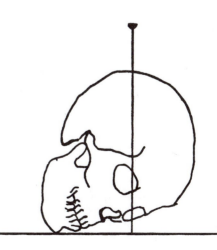

▶ STUDY QUESTIONS

1. List the 14 facial bones:

   _____

   _____

   _____

   _____

   _____

   _____

   _____

   _____

   _____

   _____

   _____

   _____

   _____

   _____

2. The right and left _____ are the largest immovable bones of the face.

3. The _____ bones are L-shaped, having both vertical and horizontal plates.

4. The prominence of the cheek is formed by the _____ _____ bone.

5. The _____ bones are small bones located in the anterior part of the medial orbital wall.

6. The bridge of the nose is formed by the right and left _____ bones.

7. The _____ are scroll-shaped facial bones demonstrated within the nasal fossa on a PA projection of the skull.

8. The _____ forms the inferior and posterior portion of the bony nasal septum.

9. The only movable facial bone is the U-shaped _____ _____ .

10. The maxillary sinuses are contained within the _____ _____ of the maxillae.

11. The _____ is a small hole on each maxilla just under the lower margin of the orbit.

12. The superior orbital fissure is formed between the _____ and _____ of the _____ bone.

13. The inferior orbital fissure is located within the floor of the orbit and is formed between the _____ _____ and the _____ _____ .

14. The _____ process of the maxilla is situated between the lateral margin of the nose and the medial margin of the orbit.

15. The upper teeth are embedded in the _____ process of the maxilla.

16. The anterior three-fourths of the hard palate is formed by the _____ process of the maxillae.

17. The _____ process extends laterally from the body of the maxilla to articulate with the malar bone.

18. The tear ducts are associated with the _____ bones.

19. The posterior aspect of the hard palate is formed by the horizontal portion of the _____ bones.

20. The nasal bones articulate with the frontal bone to form the _____ suture, which corresponds to the positioning landmark known as the _____ _____ .

21. Another name for the zygomatic bone is the _____ _____ bone.

22. A type of injury in which the zygomatic bone becomes detached from the frontal, maxillary, and temporal bones is called a/an _____ fracture.

23. The lacrimal bone is located in the medial wall of the orbit adjacent to the _____ anteriorly, _____ posteriorly, and the _____ _____ superiorly.

24. The inferior nasal conchae attach to the walls of the _____ bones and extend medially into the nasal cavity.

25. The inferior surface of the vomer articulates with the

_____ .

26. The partition that divides the nasal cavity into right and left sides is known as the _____ .

27. The right and left halves of the mandible meet at a small, vertical ridge called the _____ .

28. The two vertical portions of the mandible are called

_____ .

29. The word _____ refers to the chin.

30. The midpoint of the flat, triangular area on the chin is a positioning landmark known as the _____

_____ .

31. Where are the mental foramina located? _____

_____

32. The angle of the mandible is called the _____

_____ .

33. The _____ is a concave depression located between the two processes on the superior part of the mandibular ramus.

34. The _____ is the anterior process on the mandibular ramus.

35. The rounded head or _____ of the mandible articulates with the mandibular fossa of the temporal bone to form the temporomandibular joint.

36. The temporomandibular joints are classified functionally as _____ joints with _____ _____ type of movement.

37. The _____ bone is located at the base of the tongue between the mandible and larynx in the anterior portion of the neck.

38. The base of the orbit is formed by the _____ , _____ , and _____ bones.

39. Name the seven bones that contribute to the composition of each orbit.

_____

_____

_____

_____

_____

_____

_____

40. The circular opening at the apex of the orbit is known as the _____ .

41. Each cone-shaped orbit projects _____ ° (degrees) superiorly and _____ ° (degrees) medially into the skull.

42. When a blow-out fracture occurs, which part of the orbit is injured? _____

_____

43. What radiographic projection will best demonstrate a blow-out fracture? _____

_____

44. The joints formed by the articulation of the teeth with the bony sockets of the maxillae and mandible are known as _____ .

45. The only two synovial joints in the cranium are the _____ and _____ .

46. When a person opens his or her mouth, the condyle of the mandible moves _____ (backward/forward) in the fossa.

47. The _____ sinuses are located behind a person's forehead, specifically behind the glabella.

48. The _____ sinuses are also known as the antra of Highmore.

49. The _____ sinuses are located directly below the sella turcica.

50. The _____ sinuses consist of three groups of air cells located between the nasal cavity and each orbit.

51. If an individual has an infection affecting the maxillary sinuses, why might he complain that his teeth hurt? _____ _____

52. How does the radiographer determine which lateral projection should be taken as part of a routine facial bone series? _____ _____

53. Why should radiography of the paranasal sinuses be performed with the patient in the erect position? _____ _____

54. The _____ is a tomographic technique used for radiography of the mandible.

55. To project the petrous ridges into the lower one-third of the orbits on a PA projection of the facial bones, the central ray is angled _____ (degree and direction).

56. On a PA projection of the paranasal sinuses, the central ray is directed to the level of _____ .

57. The maxillary sinuses are best demonstrated on the _____ _____ projection.

58. Name the paranasal sinuses that are best demonstrated on a PA projection. _____ _____

59. What is the centering point for a lateral projection of the paranasal sinuses? _____ _____

60. When the radiographer is positioning a patient for a submentovertical projection of the paranasal sinuses, the _____ line should be parallel to the film plane.

61. To demonstrate the superior orbital fissures on a PA projection, the central ray should be angled _____ _____ (degree and direction).

62. On a parietoacanthial (Waters) projection of the facial bones, the central ray is directed to the level of _____ _____ .

63. On a PA projection of the facial bones for the mandibular rami, the central ray is directed perpendicular to the film at the level of _____ .

64. The infraorbitomeatal line (IOML) forms a _____ ° (degree) angle to the film plane on a parietoacanthial (Waters) projection.

65. To modify the parietoacanthial projection to better demonstrate the lower rim of the orbit, the head is tilted to place the infraorbitomeatal line (IOML) at a _____ ° (degree) angle to the film plane.

66. Where will you see the coronoid processes of the mandible on a parietoacanthial projection of the facial bones? _____ _____

67. You are positioning a patient for a lateral projection of the facial bones. Which lines/planes will you use to ensure correct positioning? _____ _____

68. You are viewing a parietoacanthial projection of the facial bones. What structures will you look at to determine if the IOML was positioned accurately? How can you determine if rotation is present on the radiograph? _____ _____ _____ _____

69. On a parieto-orbital oblique (Rhese) projection for the right optic foramen, the midsagittal plane forms an angle of _____ ° (degrees) to the film plane with the _____ (left/right) side of the head positioned closest to the table.

70. What radiographic projection can be taken to best demonstrate the zygomatic arches bilaterally? _____ _____

71. On a tangential projection of the left zygomatic arch, the head is rotated _____ ° (degrees) _____ (away from/toward) the side of interest and the central ray is directed perpendicular to the _____ line.

72. The PA axial projection of the mandibular condyles requires a _____ (degree and direction) angulation of the central ray.

73. To demonstrate the body of the mandible on an axiolateral oblique projection, the head should be rotated approximately _____ ° (degrees) toward the film and the central ray directed approximately _____ _____ (degree and direction).

74. You are viewing a closed-mouth axiolateral oblique projection of the right temporomandibular joint. If the left TMJ is included in the collimated field, where will it be seen on the radiograph? (Describe its location relative to the right TMJ.) _____ _____

75. Complete the following table:

Projection	CR Angle/Angle of Part	Centering Point	Film Size	Structures Seen
PA sinuses				
SMV for zygomatic arches				
Parietoacanthial (Waters) for facial bones				
Left lateral nasal bones				
Right axiolateral temporo-mandibular joint				

► CASE STUDIES

1. A comatose patient in the intensive care unit has spiked a fever. Her physicians are concerned that the fever is the result of a bacterial sinus infection and have ordered a sinus series to be done at the bedside. The supine patient is intubated and is unable to sit up or roll over.

   ► Discuss what projections you must take to complete a sinus series and how you will obtain them.

   ► Explain how this portable sinus series can be done to visualize possible air–fluid levels in the sinuses that would indicate sinusitis.

   ► Describe how sinusitis would visualize on the radiographs.

2. A female patient has been brought to the emergency department following a severe beating. A facial series has been requested, including bilateral zygomatic arches. The patient has several abrasions on her face and her nose is bleeding. She is transported on a stretcher and is unable to sit or stand up.

   ▶ Discuss the projections you will take for the basic facial series and the method of obtaining the radiographs.

   ▶ Describe how you will visualize the zygomatic arches.

   ▶ Discuss the precautions necessary to take regarding the patient's wounds.

1. Define the term "contrast medium." _____
   _____

2. Why are contrast media routinely employed for radiographic examinations of the digestive and urinary systems? _____
   _____

3. Negative contrast media are _____ (radiolucent/radiopaque).

4. Give an example of a common negative contrast agent. _____
   _____

5. Explain how a negative contrast medium is used routinely in chest radiography. _____
   _____

6. A positive contrast agent absorbs _____ (more / less) radiation than a negative contrast agent.

7. Give an example of a positive contrast medium commonly used for radiography of the alimentary canal. _____

8. The atomic number of iodine is _____ (lower / higher) than the atomic number of oxygen; therefore, it appears _____ (lighter / darker) on a radiograph.

9. Why should barium sulfate *never* be administered intravascularly?
   _____

10. The weight-to-volume (W/V) ratio represents the concentration of in the contrast _____ medium solution.

11. An iodinated contrast agent with a _____ (low / high) W/V ratio is used for urography, while a _____ (low / high) W/V ratio is generally used for arteriography.

12. An oil-based iodinated contrast medium is _____ (soluble / insoluble) in body fluids.

13. Oil-based iodinated contrast media are used primarily for radiography of the _____.

14. Identify a characteristic of an oil-based iodinated contrast medium that may be an advantage during radiography,but is also considered to be a disadvantage.
   _____
   _____

13

INTRODUCTION TO CONTRAST STUDIES

15. What does the term "water soluble" mean with regard to contrast media? _____

_____

16. A benzene ring contains _____ atoms of iodine per molecule.

17. A water-soluble iodinated contrast medium is usually excreted by the _____ within _____ hours after intravascular administration.

18. The concentration of charged particles in a solution per kilogram of water is known as _____ .

19. A/an _____ is a negatively charged particle, while a/an _____ is a positively charged particle.

20. How does a nonionic contrast medium differ from an ionic contrast medium? _____

_____

21. What is the element in a nonionic water-soluble contrast agent that causes it to be radiopaque? _____

_____

22. How is the osmolality of an injectable contrast agent related to the homeostasis of the body and physiologic reactions? _____

_____

_____

23. Identify five patient conditions that might warrant the use of a nonionic contrast medium over an ionic contrast medium:

_____

_____

_____

_____

_____

24. The radiographer should check the name of the contrast medium at least _____ times prior to administration.

25. A 2-year-old child is scheduled for an excretory urogram. Who determines the dosage of the contrast medium to be administered? _____

26. What criteria determine the route of administration of a contrast medium? _____

_____

_____

27. What are the acceptable routes of administration for barium sulfate contrast media? _____

_____

28. In excretory urography, an iodinated contrast medium is administered via the _____ route.

29. Name a radiographic examination in which a contrast medium is administered directly to the anatomy of interest. _____

30. According to the Chemotoxic Theory, why do more adverse reactions occur after intravascular injection than oral administration of iodinated contrast media? _____

_____

31. A/an _____ reaction resembles a true allergic reaction and the patient demonstrates hypersensitivity when the contrast medium is injected.

32. During intravenous injection, contrast media can seep into surrounding tissues if the needle is incorrectly placed in the vein. This condition is known as _____

_____ .

33. A patient who is extremely anxious about the injection of contrast media or the examination in general may experience a/an _____ reaction.

34. What are the three classifications of adverse reactions that can occur upon the administration of contrast media? _____ , _____ ,

_____

35. Which classification of contrast media reactions is considered to be life-threatening? _____

36. Which classification of contrast media reactions is considered to be self-limiting? _____

37. A skin reaction in which the patient develops a few hives is known as _____ .

38. What information regarding a contrast study should the radiographer discuss with the patient prior to the administration of a contrast medium? _____
_____
_____

39. List several supplies that should be available in the radiographic room prior to the start of a procedure using contrast media. _____
_____
_____

40. Imagine that you are a patient scheduled for an upper GI examination. As you are transported into the radiography room, you noticed that the room seems cluttered and there are barium stains on the pillowcase. What nonverbal message does the condition of the room convey to you? _____
_____
_____

41. As the radiographer scheduled in a fluoroscopic room, describe how you will prepare the room for an upper GI examination. _____
_____
_____
_____

42. When setting up the control panel for a fluoroscopic examination, the fluoroscopic timer should be set at _____ minutes.

43. A young infant is immobilized on an octagon board in preparation for an upper GI examination. As the radiographer scheduled in the room, you must stand at the head of the table to assist the radiologist in positioning the infant. How can you minimize your exposure to scatter radiation? _____
_____

44. A patient is scheduled to have the following series of tests performed. Arrange them in the order in which they should be performed for optimum results: UGI, ultrasound of the gallbladder, and oral cholecystogram.

A _____

B _____

C _____

45. Is it possible to perform both an excretory urogram and a barium enema on a patient on the same day? Explain your answer. _____
_____

INDICATE *TRUE* OR *FALSE* FOR QUESTIONS 46–50.

46. _____ Iodinated contrast media are available in a variety of forms for oral, rectal, intravascular, or direct administration.

47. _____ A double contrast examination of the large intestine would require the use of both water-soluble iodinated and barium sulfate contrast media.

48. _____ Radiographers are licensed to dispense contrast media but not any other type of pharmaceutical.

49. _____ When an iodinated contrast medium is administered intravenously, it is usually injected into a vein on the anterior surface of the elbow or on the dorsum of the hand.

50. _____ According to the Chemotoxic Theory, the amount of contrast medium and the speed at which it is injected are factors relating to the occurrence of adverse reactions.

► WORD SEARCH

USING THE FOLLOWING CLUES, FIND TERMI-
NOLOGY RELATED TO CONTRAST MEDIA IN
THE WORD SEARCH PUZZLE.

1. Resembles an allergic reaction

2. A reaction brought on by fear or anxiety

3. A drug, including contrast agents

4. Condition of fluid overload in the circulatory system

5. Maintenance of constant conditions within the body

6. Reaction caused by contrast medium seeping out of the vein during intravenous injection

7. Sweating profusely

8. A concentrated amount of contrast media is injected over a short period of time

9. The degree to which a contrast agent is poisonous

10. Concerning the movement of blood within the circulatory system

11. An iodinated contrast medium that separates into charged particles

12. Contrast medium is diluted with sterile water and slowly administered intravenously

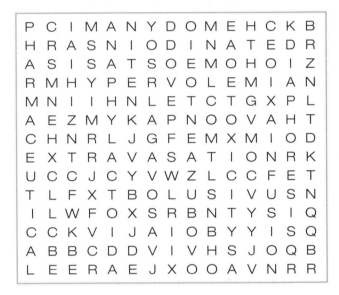

```
P  C  I  M  A  N  Y  D  O  M  E  H  C  K  B
H  R  A  S  N  I  O  D  I  N  A  T  E  D  R
A  S  I  S  A  T  S  O  E  M  O  H  O  I  Z
R  M  H  Y  P  E  R  V  O  L  E  M  I  A  N
M  N  I  I  H  N  L  E  T  C  T  G  X  P  L
A  E  Z  M  Y  K  A  P  N  O  O  V  A  H  T
C  H  N  R  L  J  G  F  E  M  X  M  I  O  D
E  X  T  R  A  V  A  S  A  T  I  O  N  R  K
U  C  C  J  C  Y  V  W  Z  L  C  C  F  E  T
T  L  F  X  T  B  O  L  U  S  I  V  U  S  N
I  L  W  F  O  X  S  R  B  N  T  Y  S  I  Q
C  C  K  V  I  J  A  I  O  B  Y  Y  I  S  Q
A  B  B  C  D  D  V  I  V  H  S  J  O  Q  B
L  E  E  R  A  E  J  X  O  O  A  V  N  R  R
```

1. List the components of the urinary system: _____
   _____
   _____

2. Name the organ(s) responsible for producing urine. _____

3. Describe the role of the urinary system in maintaining the homeostasis of the
   body. _____
   _____
   _____

4. Describe the location of the kidneys in relationship to the vertebral column.
   _____
   _____

5. Due to the presence of the _____ muscles, the kidneys rest
   obliquely at an angle of _____ ° (degrees).

6. Are the kidneys located more *anteriorly* or *posteriorly* in the abdomen?
   _____

7. The kidneys are tilted posteriorly at an angle of _____ ° (degrees) to the midsagittal plane.

8. Which kidney lies more inferiorly in the abdominal cavity? Explain
   your answer.? _____
   _____

9. The ureter leaves the kidney at a deep fissure on the medial border called the
   _____ .

10. What are the *poles* of the kidney? _____
    _____

11. The _____ of the kidney is also
    known as the perirenal fat.

12. What is the *renal parenchyma?* _____
    _____

13. The nephrons are located primarily in the _____
    of the kidney.

14. Where is the fibrous renal capsule located? _____
    _____

14

URINARY SYSTEM

15. What characteristic of the kidneys allows the renal shadows to be demonstrated on a radiograph without contrast media? _____ _____

16. The pointed apices or _____ of the renal pyramids project inward toward the renal sinus.

17. There are approximately _____ renal pyramids located in the _____ of the kidney.

18. The _____ and _____ are tubelike branches of the renal pelvis, which channel the urine in from the pyramids.

19. Bundles of collecting tubules primarily form the triangular _____ of the kidney.

20. The expanded medial portion of the renal pelvis continues as the _____ .

21. The _____ functions to store urine until it can be eliminated from the body.

22. The physiologic or functional element of the kidney is the _____ .

23. Approximately 50 intertwining capillaries form a ball-like cluster called the _____ .

24. List the three main functions performed by the nephron. _____ _____ _____

25. The cup-shaped _____ surrounds the glomerulus and absorbs substances filtered from it.

26. What is the *renal corpuscle?* _____ _____

27. How is the glomerulus able to filter wastes, water, salts, and sugar out of the bloodstream? _____ _____

28. The basic composition of urine is _____ % water and _____ % solid waste substances such as urea, creatinine, and salts.

29. On the average, approximately how many liters of urine does a person produce daily? _____

30. Vital salts, nutrients, and water filter out of the _____ _____ of the nephron and are reabsorbed by the bloodstream.

31. A/an _____ supplies each kidney with oxygenated blood.

32. The terms _____ and _____ _____ refer to a kidney stone.

33. What is the function of the ureters? _____ _____

34. The ureterovesical junction is located on the _____ _____ aspect of the urinary bladder.

35. The muscular layer of tissue comprising the ureter permits rhythmic contractions called _____ which help convey the urine to the urinary bladder.

36. Kidney stones are likely to lodge in the following three areas of constriction along the ureter:

_____

_____

_____

37. _____ is a method of treating kidney stones by using sound waves to shatter them.

38. The urinary bladder is an expandable sac located directly behind the _____ and directly anterior to the _____ on a female.

39. Describe the location of the kidneys, ureters, and urinary bladder in relationship to the parietal peritoneum. _____ _____ _____

40. When the urinary bladder is empty, its mucosal lining falls into folds known as _____ .

41. The _____ is a smooth, triangular area on the floor of the urinary bladder.

42. _____ is defined as the act of voiding or urinating.

43. Involuntary urination is known as _____ _____ .

44. The hollow tube leading from the urinary bladder to the exterior of the body is the _____ .

45. The three corners of the trigone in the urinary bladder are formed by the: _____ and _____ .

46. The male urethra functions in both the urinary and _____ systems.

47. An inflammation of the urinary bladder is known as _____ .

48. _____ is a general term referring to radiography of the urinary system.

49. The _____ is the opening of the urethra to the outside of the body.

50. Explain why an excretory urogram is considered to be a functional examination of the urinary system. _____ _____ _____ _____

51. Radiographs of the kidneys taken soon after injection of contrast media are called _____ .

52. Explain the reason for performing a hypertensive excretory urogram (IVP) on a patient. _____ _____

53. Why should a patient's creatinine level be checked prior to performing an excretory urogram? _____ _____

54. Identify a nonfunctional examination that may be performed to evaluate the renal pelvis, calyces, and ureter when an excretory urogram is contraindicated. _____ _____

55. Define *vesicoureteral reflux*. What examinations will demonstrate it radiographically? _____ _____

56. What nonfunctional radiographic examination will demonstrate the shape and position of the urinary bladder after the introduction of contrast medium through a catheter? _____

57. Name the only radiographic examination of the urinary system that will demonstrate the urethra. _____ _____

58. What is the purpose of giving a patient a cathartic (laxative) on the evening prior to an excretory urogram? _____ _____ _____

59. You have to perform an excretory urogram on a patient with a urinary catheter. Discuss what you will do with the catheter and collection bag during the procedure. _____ _____ _____

60. Timing during an excretory urogram begins at the _____ _____ (start / completion) of the injection of contrast medium.

61. Oblique projections of the kidneys during an excretory urogram require that the patient be rotated _____ ° (degrees) from an AP position.

62. When the patient is rotated to an LPO position, the _____ _____ kidney is parallel to the film plane.

63. What is the purpose of using a ureteral compression device? _____ _____

64. What type of contrast medium is employed in urography? _____

65. What is the advantage of using tomography during an excretory urogram? _____ _____

66. Why is a young child often given a carbonated beverage during an excretory urogram? _____ _____

67. The recommended breathing instructions for urography are _____ _____ .

68. A radiograph taken 10 minutes after injection during an excretory urogram would routinely be taken on a/an _____ in. (size) film and centered to the level of _____ .

69. Where would the radiographer direct the central ray to localize the kidneys on a nephrogram? _____ _____

70. What is the recommended range of kVp for urography? Explain your answer. _____ _____

71. On an AP oblique projection of the urinary bladder, the patient will be rotated _____ ° (degrees) from an AP position.

72. Which ureterovesical junction would be best demonstrated if the patient was placed in the right posterior oblique position? _____

73. How can rotation be detected on an AP projection of the urinary bladder? _____ _____

74. On an AP projection of the urinary bladder, the central ray is directed _____ (degree and direction) to the point _____ .

75. Complete the following table:

Projection	CR Angle/Angle of Part	Centering Point	Film Size	Structures Seen
AP urinary tract post-injection				
LPO urinary bladder				
RPO urinary tract				

ACROSS

3. Involuntary urination
6. Presence of blood in the urine
9. Inflammation of the urinary bladder
10. Toxic build-up of nitrogenous waste materials in the blood
11. Excision of the kidney
12. Tubelike structures that branch off of the renal pelvis
13. Scanty urine output
14. Procedure that artificially filters and cleans the blood in an individual with kidney failure
15. Examination performed to evaluate renal function; also known as an excretory urogram
16. Location of the urinary bladder in the abdominopelvic cavity
17. Malposition of the kidneys, as in the case of pelvic kidneys

DOWN

1. The act of urinating
2. Prolapse or downward displacement of the kidney
4. Introduction of a flexible, rubber tube into the urinary bladder via the urethra to remove urine
5. Kidney stone
7. Laboratory procedure in which the components of urine are analyzed
8. Abnormal condition in which urine is not being produced
9. An instrument with a light source that is used to visually examine the urinary bladder
11. The microscopic, functional unit of the kidney

▶ CASE STUDY

1. A 48-year-old male patient has been transported to the Radiology Department by stretcher for an intravenous urogram. He has a urinary catheter in place. He tells you that he is in extreme pain and is unable to move by himself. The patient's body habitus is hypersthenic as he is approximately 6 ft 7 in. tall and weighs about 300 pounds.

   ▶ Discuss the procedure you will use to move this patient to the radiographic table since he is unable to do so by himself.

   ▶ How will you handle the urinary collection bag during the radiographic procedure?

   ▶ Discuss the questions that should be asked when obtaining a patient history.

   ▶ After injection of the contrast medium, the patient begins to itch. Upon examination, you notice several small hives on his neck and face. How would you classify this reaction? How would it be treated?

   ▶ The radiologist requests a collimated AP projection of the kidneys. Describe how you will localize the kidneys on this patient.

   ▶ A nephrolith is suspected in the region of the right ureterovesical junction. What projection could you take to best demonstrate this area?

   ....

   ....

   ....

   ....

   ....

   ....

   ....

   ....

   ....

► STUDY QUESTIONS

1. The continuous hollow tube of the digestive system is known as the gastrointestinal tract or _____.

2. List the accessory organs of digestion: _____
_____

3. The inner layer of tissue lining the walls of the gastrointestinal tract is called the _____.

4. The mouth is also known as the oral or _____ cavity.

5. What part of the oral cavity is formed by the soft and hard palates? _____
_____

6. Explain the role of the tongue in the process of digestion. _____
_____

7. The process of chewing is known as _____.

8. The opening between the oral cavity and the oropharynx is called the _____
_____

9. The _____ (hard / soft) palate is a musculomembranous fold of tissue that acts as a partition between the mouth and pharynx.

10. The largest of the salivary glands, known as the _____ glands, are located in the cheeks.

11. How do the teeth aid in the digestive process? _____
_____

12. Name the three pairs of salivary glands. _____
_____
_____

13. Define *deglutition.* _____

14. Describe the location of the sublingual glands. _____
_____

15. When a person swallows a bolus of food, what prevents it from entering the larynx instead of the esophagus? _____
_____

16. What is the approximate length of the esophagus?
_____

17. The esophagus begins approximately at the level of the _____ vertebra and ends at the level of the _____ vertebra.

18. What is the function of the esophagus? _____ _____

19. As the esophagus passes into the abdominopelvic cavity, it passes through an opening in the diaphragm known as the _____ , which is located at the level of the _____ vertebra.

20. The short abdominal segment of the esophagus is also referred to as the _____ as it is located near the heart.

21. The esophagogastric junction is located at the level of the _____ vertebra.

22. The mucosal lining of the stomach falls into folds called _____ when the stomach is empty.

23. The _____ orifice is the opening where the esophagus enters the stomach.

24. _____ is a semifluid pastelike substance that results from the churning of food in the stomach.

25. List the three main portions of the stomach. _____ _____ _____

26. As fluids and food substances leave the stomach, they pass through the _____ orifice into the small intestine.

27. The upper, rounded portion of the stomach is the _____ _____ .

28. What is the role of the pyloric sphincter? _____ _____

29. Which curvature is located on the lateral margin of the stomach? _____

30. The _____ notch is located on the lesser curvature of the stomach between the body and pyloric antrum.

31. Describe the location and shape of the stomach on an asthenic patient. _____ _____

32. On expiration, the stomach moves _____ (inferiorly / superiorly) in the abdominopelvic cavity.

33. Which portion of the digestive tract is arch-shaped and is generally positioned around the periphery of the abdominopelvic cavity? _____

34. List the segments of the small intestine in the correct sequence. _____ _____

35. Which segment of the small intestine is the longest? _____

36. In which quadrant of the abdomen is the duodenojejunal flexure located? _____

37. Which segment of the small intestine is primarily located in the middle and lower right regions of the abdomen? _____

38. Which segment of the small intestine is the largest in diameter? _____

39. The terminal ileum is generally located in the _____ _____ quadrant of the abdomen.

40. Small circular fold in the mucous membrane of the small intestine are known as _____ .

41. After the oral administration of barium sulfate, which segment of the small intestine will appear light and feathery on a radiograph? _____

42. The saclike region at the beginning of the large intestine is the _____ .

43. The appendix is also known as the _____ _____ and is usually located in the _____ quadrant of the abdomen.

44. You are viewing an AP projection of the abdomen taken after the rectal administration of barium sulfate. Describe specifically where you would expect the descending colon to be demonstrated. _____ _____

45. The S-shaped portion of the large intestine is called the _____ .

46. The bend in the large intestine between the ascending colon and the transverse colon is known as the_____ _____ .

47. The dilated portion of the rectum located just anterior to the coccyx is known as the _____ .

48. The _____ are three bands of longitudinal muscle that extend the length of the large intestine except at the rectum.

49. Which of the flexures of the colon extends more superiorly than the other? _____

50. Characteristically, the large intestine has sacs or pouches called _____ , which result from the presence of the longitudinal bands of muscle.

51. What role does the liver play in the digestive process? _____

52. Once bile is released by the gallbladder, it enters which region of the alimentary canal? _____

53. How does the pancreas aid in digestion? _____ _____

54. Explain why respiration is temporarily suspended for 1–3 seconds during deglutition. _____ _____ _____

55. Food is propelled through portions of the alimentary canal by a series of wavelike contractions known as _____ .

56. Organic catalysts that expedite chemical digestion are called _____ .

57. In which region of the alimentary canal do the majority of digestive and absorptive processes take place? _____ _____

58. _____ refers to the process of eliminating feces from the large intestine.

59. On the average, how long does it take for chyme to pass completely through the small intestine? _____ _____

60. Barium sulfate that is administered orally will take approximately _____ hours to pass from the mouth to the anus.

61. Once water is absorbed from chyme in the large intestine, a semisolid material known as _____ is formed.

62. A barium swallow exam would be performed to evaluate which region of the alimentary canal? _____ _____

63. To diagnose Crohn's disease, which region of the alimentary canal would most likely be examined? _____ _____

64. Explain how and why the patient preparation for an esophagram differs from the preparation for an upper GI examination. _____ _____ _____ _____

65. Describe the type of contrast media administered in a double-contrast barium enema. _____ _____

66. Examination of the salivary ducts following the injection of iodinated contrast medium is known as _____ _____ .

67. An examination of the small intestine in which contrast medium is injected via a long tube is called _____ _____ .

68. Recommended breathing instructions for radiographic examinations of the alimentary canal are _____ _____ .

69. Describe the instructions given to the patient for the Valsalva maneuver _____ _____ .

70. On an AP projection of the esophagus, the central ray should be directed perpendicular to the level of _____ _____.

71. Why are breathing instructions unnecessary when the patient is continuously swallowing barium sulfate for projections of the esophagus?_____ _____

72. On an RAO projection of the esophagus, the patient should be rotated approximately _____ ° (degrees), with an asthenic patient being rotated _____ (less / more) than a hypersthenic patient.

73. What is the purpose of performing the toe touch exercise (maneuver) during an esophagram?_____ _____

74. When positioning a patient for a lateral projection of the esophagus, which plane or line is centered longitudinally to the midline of the table? _____

75. Identify the projection that best demonstrates the barium-filled esophagus by placing it between the spine and the heart. _____

76. For a PA projection of the stomach on a sthenic patient, the central ray will be directed to the _____ _____ , which is at the level of the _____ vertebra.

77. Describe how centering of the PA projection of the stomach would change for a hypersthenic patient._____ _____ _____

78. Would the fundus of the stomach be filled with air or barium sulfate on an AP projection?_____ _____

79. On an RAO projection of the stomach, the patient's coronal plane should form an angle of_____ ° (degrees) to the table.

80. When positioning a hypersthenic patient for an RAO projection of the stomach, the patient must be obliqued _____ (less / more) than a sthenic patient.

81. Which projection will best demonstrate the anterior and posterior surfaces of the stomach? _____ _____

82. Which projection(s) would you take to best demonstrate the greater and lesser curvature of the stomach?_____ _____

83. Which projection of the stomach will best demonstrate the duodenal bulb and C-loop in profile and free of superimposition by the pylorus?_____

84. You are viewing a lateral projection of the stomach. How will you evaluate it for rotation?_____ _____

85. Complete this statement relative to positioning for an LPO projection of the stomach: center the longitudinal plane passing _____ to the midline of the table.

86. What is the purpose of using a time marker on an AP or PA projection of the small bowel?_____ _____

87. When is a small bowel series considered to be complete? _____ _____

88. On an AP projection of the large intestine, the central ray is directed perpendicular to the level of _____ _____.

89. You just completed a double-contrast barium enema and are now viewing the patient's radiographs. The transverse colon will be filled with _____ on the AP projection and with _____ on the PA projection.

90. Referring to the study in the previous question, the ascending colon and descending colon are located _____ (anteriorly/posteriorly) and will fill with barium sulfate when the patient is supine.

91. Which oblique projection(s) will best demonstrate the right colic (hepatic) flexure, ascending colon, and the cecum?_____

92. For the anterior or posterior oblique projections of the large intestine, the patient should be rotated approximately _____ ° (degrees).

93. What is the purpose of taking a "scout" radiograph prior to fluoroscopy of the alimentary canal?_____ _____

94. To demonstrate the rectosigmoid region of the large intestine on an AP axial projection, the central ray should be directed _____ (degree and direction) to the level of _____ when a 14 × 17-in. cassette is used.

95. You are viewing a radiograph of the small intestine taken 60 minutes after the administration of barium sulfate. You note that the ileum is much smoother in appearance than the jejunum. What is the reason for the different appearance of the ileum and jejunum radiographically?_____ _____ _____

96. If the rectosigmoid area is still superimposed on an AP axial projection, which oblique projection could be taken to better demonstrate the area?_____ _____

97. The radiologist would like to evaluate polyps on the lateral aspect of a patient's descending colon. Which decubitus projection can you take to demonstrate this area filled with air on a double-contrast examination? _____

98. On which projection of the large intestine will the rectum be demonstrated in profile and anterior to the sacrum? _____

99. What is the centering point for a lateral projection of the rectum when a 10 × 12-in. cassette is used? _____ _____

100. Complete the following table:

Projection	CR Angle/Angle of Part	Centering Point	Film Size	Structures Seen
RAO esophagus				
Right lateral stomach				
RPO large intestine				
Left lateral rectum				

▶ WORD SEARCH

USING THE FOLLOWING CLUES, FIND TERMI-
NOLOGY RELATED TO THE DIGESTIVE SYSTEM
IN THE WORD SEARCH PUZZLE.

1. Inflammation of the appendix

2. Inflammatory condition of the colon

3. Difficulty in eliminating fecal material

4. Inflammatory bowel condition usually affecting the small intestine

5. Sacs or pouches protruding outward from the walls of the alimentary canal

6. Intestinal gas, usually expelled through the anus

7. Inflammatory condition of the stomach

8. Dilated veins in the rectum, particularly in the anal canal

9. Small bowel obstruction

10. Telescoping of one area of intestine into the lumen of the adjacent area

11. Infectious condition in which one or both parotid glands are inflamed

12. Sick feeling that may result in vomiting

13. Abnormal growth on the mucous membrane of a structure; may protrude into the lumen of the alimentary canal

14. Hernia or prolapse of the rectum

15. Hollow or craterlike lesion on the mucous membrane of a structure

16. Condition in which a loop of intestine twists, resulting in an obstruction

```
B U F E G A S T R I T I S X N
L S W L V S N T T Q Y R D O D
W N A U S E A T M M N A I D B
D V O L V U L U S R W T O E N
S I T I C I D N E P P A H X J
V P V K T I I C O E O T R P G
W O M E I A L X C M K X R J S
C Q Y U R U P S K B G O O J M
V R C S M T U I D X C G M E F
O A O W M S I P T T I L E U S
I W L H S B K C O S S F H Y H
L A I U N T D C U L N O G A C
B D T L S S E V Q L Y O Y W M
P N I N F L A T U S A P C Y F
I K S L E T I Z S D U H S E E
```

▶ CASE STUDIES

1. A 2-week-old infant has been brought to the imaging department by his parents for an esophagram. The possible diagnosis is esophageal atresia.

   ▶ How will the infant be immobilized during the procedure?

   ▶ Describe the use of any special equipment needed for the procedure.

   ▶ How will the contrast medium be administered to the infant?

   ▶ Discuss the patient preparation that was necessary for this exam.

   ▶ How will esophageal atresia be visualized on the radiographs?

   ▶ Discuss the use of lead shielding for the infant, as well as for any person assisting in the procedure.

2. A barium enema has been ordered on a 68-year-old male patient with a colostomy. The procedure is being performed to evaluate the large intestine prior to surgery to reverse the colostomy. The patient states that he is able to move well, but cannot lie on his abdomen.

> ▸ Discuss the questions that should be asked when obtaining a patient history.

> ▸ Routine overhead projections for a barium enema include a PA axial projection of the sigmoid colon. Describe how you will obtain an axial projection of the sigmoid colon on this patient.

> ▸ What special precautions must you take during the procedure?

► STUDY QUESTIONS

1. Identify the structures of the biliary system. _____
_____

2. In which quadrant of the abdomen is the liver primarily located? _____
_____

3. Describe the location of the liver in relationship to the diaphragm. _____
_____

4. The liver is divided into _____ lobes.

5. The _____ separates the right and left lobes
and helps suspend the liver from the diaphragm.

6. Liver cells are known as _____ .

7. What is a liver lobule? _____
_____

8. The _____ are tiny bile capillaries that form a network of
ducts around the liver cells.

9. The portal vein and hepatic artery enter the liver at a transverse fissure on its
posteroinferior surface known as the _____
or hilus of the liver.

10. What function does bile perform in the process of digestion? _____
_____

11. The minor lobes of the liver are known as the _____
and _____ lobes.

12. Which organ of the biliary system produces bile? _____
_____

13. The gallbladder lies on the _____ surface of the liver.

14. On the sthenic individual, the gallbladder is usually located at the level of
the _____ costal cartilage.

15. List the three main parts of the gallbladder:
_____ , _____
_____

16. To localize the gallbladder on a hypersthenic patient, the radiographer must
center _____(higher / lower) and more _____
(medially / laterally) than on the sthenic patient.

17. When a person is viewed from the side, the gallbladder is _____
_____ (anterior / posterior) to the midcoronal plane of the body.

BILIARY SYSTEM

18. What is the main function of the gallbladder? _____
_____

19. What characteristic of the gallbladder enables it to contract and expand? _____
_____

20. The _____ of the gallbladder is its rounded distal portion.

21. Bile enters and leaves the gallbladder via the _____
_____ duct.

22. Define *cholelith.* _____
_____

23. Bile is drained from the major lobes of the liver by the _____ ducts.

24. The _____ duct and _____
_____ duct merge to form the common bile duct.

25. The hormone _____
is secreted by the mucosal lining of the duodenum and prompts the gallbladder to contract and expel bile.

26. Before entering the duodenum, the common bile duct and pancreatic duct merge to form the _____
_____ .

27. Define emulsification as it relates to the biliary system.
_____

28. What are the duodenal papillae?
_____

29. Describe the location of the pancreas in relationship to the duodenum. _____
_____

30. Two hormones that are secreted by the pancreas and play a role in the metabolism of carbohydrates are _____ and _____ .

31. Which part of the pancreas lies in close proximity to the spleen? _____
_____

32. Radiography of the gallbladder is known as _____
_____ .

33. Radiographic examination of the biliary ducts is called
_____ .

34. What is a *cholecystogogue?*
_____

35. When taking a patient history prior to an oral cholecystogram, why should the patient be asked about any occurrences of vomiting or diarrhea after ingestion of the contrast medium? _____
_____

36. A general term for the iodinated contrast medium used to visualize the biliary system is _____ .

37. Which projection(s) of the gallbladder can be taken to demonstrate the stratification of stones? _____
_____

38. An asthenic patient must be rotated _____
(less / more) than a hypersthenic patient for the oblique projection of the gallbladder.

39. What is the reason for performing a postoperative or T-tube cholangiogram? _____
_____

40. What is an *ERCP?*
_____

41. Explain the reason for performing a percutaneous transhepatic cholangiogram under sterile conditions and following universal precautions. _____
_____
_____
_____

42. The recommended breathing instructions for cholecystography are _____ .

43. On an LAO position of the gallbladder, the patient should be rotated approximately _____° (degrees).

44. On a recumbent PA projection of the gallbladder using a 10 × 12-in. film, the radiographer should direct the central ray perpendicular to the level of _____
_____ on a sthenic patient.

INDICATE TRUE OR FALSE FOR QUESTIONS 45–49.

_____ 45. The pancreas plays a role in both the biliary and endocrine systems.

_____ 46. Cholecystokinin causes the hepatopancreatic sphincter to relax, allowing bile and pancreatic juice to enter the duodenum.

_____ 47. Cholesterol is a component of bile and is often a main constituent of gallstones.

_____ 48. The liver manufactures bile on an as-needed basis when a person eats fatty foods.

_____ 49. The gallbladder is relatively fixed in place behind the liver and its position in the abdomen is affected solely by a person's body habitus.

50. Complete the following table:

Projection	CR Angle/Angle of Part	Centering Point	Film Size	Structures Seen
PA upright gallbladder				
LAO gallbladder				
Right lateral decubitus gallbladder				

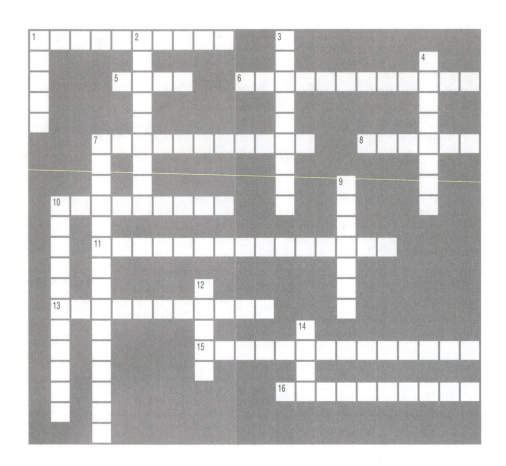

ACROSS

1. Bile enters and leaves gallbladder via this structure
5. Endoscopic examination in which the bile ducts and pancreatic duct are examined for the presence of stones or other pathology
6. Condition in which the liver is abnormally enlarged
7. Inflammation of the bile ducts
8. The rounded lower portion of the gallbladder
10. Cholelith
11. Surgical removal of the gallbladder
13. Shock wave therapy used to crush stones
15. The process of breaking down fats
16. A liver cell

DOWN

1. Root word denoting bile
2. Degenerative disease in which the liver cells are progressively destroyed
3. Inflammation of the liver
4. Yellow discoloration of the skin, usually due to a disorder of the gallbladder or liver
7. Iodinated contrast medium used in radiographic procedures of the biliary tract
9. Failure to secrete bile
10. Structure that stores and concentrates bile
12. Organ that produces bile
14. Liquid substance that helps to emulsify, absorb, and digest fats

► CASE STUDY

1. A female patient arrives in the imaging department via stretcher for an oral cholecystogram. She has been rescheduled from the previous day because her gallbladder did not visualize. She is extremely slender in build.

   ► Discuss the questions that should be asked when obtaining a patient history.

   ► She tells you that she took six pills (contrast media) on the previous evening. Although they had caused her to vomit when she took them two nights ago, she did not experience any side effects last night. How does this history relate to the nonvisualization of her gallbladder on the previous day?

   ► Describe how you will modify centering and positioning of this patient with regard to her body habitus.

   ► Since she has been recumbent for several days, she feels too weak to stand for an upright projection. What projection can you take in its place? Why is this projection necessary?

▶ STUDY QUESTIONS

1. Radiographic examination of the breast is known as _____ _____ .

2. How does the female breast differ functionally from the male breast? _____ _____ _____

3. The breast attaches to the anterior chest wall at the _____ muscle and extends from the level of the _____ to the _____ ribs.

4. The nipple is surrounded by a more pigmented area known as the _____ _____ .

5. The _____ serves as an important landmark as it is located at the convergence of the inferior aspect of the breast and the anterior chest wall.

6. The axillary tail is located in the _____ quadrant of the breast.

7. How does the location of the axillary tail of the breast relate to the spread of cancer? _____ _____ _____

8. Each breast is comprised of approximately _____ glandular lobes.

9. Dense connective tissues called _____ extend from the pectoralis major fascia to the skin anteriorly to support the weight of the breast.

10. The breast tissue of a pubescent female is categorized as _____ type.

11. The breasts of a 65-year-old mother of four are most likely composed of _____ tissue. Explain your answer. _____ _____ _____

12. The _____ category is considered to be the average type of breast tissue.

MAMMOGRAPHY

13. Which category of breast tissue is densest and therefore requires more radiographic exposure to penetrate it?

_____

14. A 55-year-old female is scheduled for a mammogram. According to her history, she had a total hysterectomy several years ago and recently began hormone replacement therapy. How would you categorize her breast tissue with regard to density? _____

_____

_____

15. What is the significance of including the pectoralis major muscle on projections of the breast? _____

_____

16. How does fibrocystic breast disease affect the density of breast tissue? _____

_____

17. Indicate whether the following are visible on a mammogram by writing *yes* or *no* in the space provided:

_____ A. skin pores

_____ B. ductal patterns

_____ C. veins

_____ D. skin thickening

_____ E. moles

18. The _____ and _____ margins of the breast are more mobile than the _____ and _____ margins.

19. The surgical removal of a breast is known as a _____

_____ .

20. A woman who has never been pregnant is described as _____ , whereas a woman who has been pregnant several times can be designated as

_____ .

21. In a procedure known as a/an _____ , a tumor is removed from the breast without the excision of surrounding breast tissue or lymph nodes.

22. _____ are minute calcium deposits in the breast that, when demonstrated on a mammogram, may indicate the presence of a malignancy.

23. What is the significance of "MSQA"? _____

_____

_____

_____

24. The American College of Radiology (ACR) recommends that the average dose for mammography not exceed _____ rad(s) per projection.

25. According to the ACS and ACR guidelines for screening mammography, at what age should a woman have her first (baseline) mammogram? _____

26. At what age should a woman begin to have yearly screening mammograms? _____

27. Why is the patient instructed to refrain from using deodorant, perfumes, or powders on the day she is having a mammogram performed? _____

_____

_____

28. Name the two localization methods used to document the location of symptoms or abnormalities on the breast.

_____

_____

29. What two projections are routinely taken for a mammogram? _____

_____

30. The radiographer wanted to use the quadrant method to record on the history form that the patient had a mole on her left breast at 5 o'clock. In which quadrant would the mole be located? _____

31. The C-arm on a dedicated mammography machine is usually rotated _____ ° (degrees) for the mediolateral oblique projection.

32. When positioning the C-arm on a mammography machine for the mediolateral oblique projection, how can the mammographer determine the correct degree of angulation that should be used for the patient? _____

_____

_____

_____

33. Why is it important that the nipple be in profile for the projections of the breast? _____

_____

34. How many pounds of pressure are routinely applied to the breast by the compression device? _____

35. A caudocranial projection of the breast is identified by a "FB" marker. What is the meaning of "FB"? _____

_____

36. Discuss the reason for taking a true 90° mediolateral or lateromedial projection of the breast in addition to the routine CC and MLO projections. _____

_____

_____

_____

37. When is the "rolled position" used in mammography? _____

_____

_____

38. When positioning the breast in the rolled position, the _____ tissue of the breast is generally rolled medially and the _____ breast tissue rolled laterally.

39. When might the radiologist request that a *cleavage projection* be performed? _____

_____

40. The radiographic examination of the collecting ducts surrounding the nipple after the injection of contrast medium is known as _____ .

41. When are magnification projections recommended? _____

_____

_____

42. Why is a needle localization procedure performed? _____

_____

_____

_____

43. Describe the projections that are routinely taken to demonstrate the augmented breast. _____

_____

_____

44. What is a stereotactic table? _____

_____

_____

45. The average range of kVp used to obtain high contrast mammograms is _____ kVp.

46. How does the mammographer select the correct photocell when using automatic exposure control? _____

_____

_____

47. The anode target on a dedicated mammography unit is usually made of _____ to produce a low energy x-ray beam for good soft tissue detail.

48. Explain how the "heel effect" is used effectively in mammography. _____

_____

_____

_____

49. Your patient tells you that compression hurts her and she prefers that you not use it. Explain the advantages of compression to her. _____

_____

_____

_____

50. According to QA guidelines and ACR recommendations, how often should intensification screens in mammography cassettes be cleaned? _____

_____

► WORD SEARCH

USING THE FOLLOWING CLUES, FIND TERMI-
NOLOGY RELATED TO MAMMOGRAPHY IN THE
WORD SEARCH PUZZLE.

1. Pigmented area surrounding the nipple
2. Pathologic examination of body tissue that has been removed from the body
3. Used to decrease the thickness of the breast tissue for better examination
4. Routine projection in which the CR is projected from the superior to the inferior aspect of the breast
5. Radiograph of the collecting ducts surrounding the nipple after injection of contrast medium
6. Milk secretion from the breast
7. Technique using increased OID to demonstrate small calcifications
8. Inflammation of breast tissue
9. Routine oblique projection
10. Projection found on the apex of the breast
11. Condition of being pregnant and delivering a child
12. Inserted into the breast to augment breast size
13. Method of localization in which breast is divided into four regions
14. Type of compression used to radiograph small area of interest in breast
15. Another name for the axillary tail of the breast

```
N O I T A C I F I N G A M G V
T L S V Q R Y T S I B S E A W
R M I L U A Q O I N I R D L U
D O T E C N E P S F O L I A T
T F I N O I S S E R P M O C P
Q L T F P O B S H A S I L T H
M L S I A C Y D T M Y M A O S
Q U A D R A N T S M S S T G A
B X M C I U T C O A L O E R A
I Q E D T D U N R R W L R A E
P C C U Y A S J P Y P R A M T
V R E S D D T P P P D U L F J
P H O B Q V P I I N K O L N S
G C R G D P G N O L J Y T L M
A R A F C X W F W N F C Q M J
```

► CASE STUDY

1. A female patient is sent to the mammography suite for a diagnostic examination. She is transported by stretcher and explains to you that she is unable to sit upright for her mammogram as she is paralyzed from the waist down.

   ► Discuss the procedure you will follow to obtain the routine projections (CC and MLO) on both breasts.

   ► The patient is very small in stature with little breast tissue. Discuss how this may affect positioning and compression.

1. The two distinct portions of the circulatory system are the _____
_____ and _____ systems.

2. _____ are the vessels that carry oxygenated blood from the heart to the tissues of the body.

3. _____ are the vessels that carry deoxygenated blood from the body back to the heart.

4. How do capillaries allow for the transfer of oxygen and nutrients to tissues and the filtration of metabolic waste products from tissues to the blood?
_____
_____
_____

5. Approximately how long does it take for blood to make a complete circuit through the body of an average individual? _____

6. List the names of the three layers of tissue forming the arterial walls.
_____
_____
_____

7. _____ circulation refers to the left ventricle of the heart and includes circulation to the entire body except the lungs.

8. In what way do the pulmonary arteries and veins differ from other arteries and veins in the body? _____
_____
_____

9. Small capillaries merge together to form the beginning branches of veins called _____ .

10. How is the movement of blood in the veins facilitated?
_____
_____

11. What is the function of the valves found within the larger veins?
_____
_____

12. Blood is pumped from the _____ of the heart through the pulmonary arteries into the lungs. Blood from the lungs returns to the _____ of the heart via the pulmonary veins.

18

CARDIOVASCULAR SYSTEM

13. The radiographic examination of the vessels of the body after the administration of iodinated contrast media is known as _____ .

14. Describe the function of the lymphatic system. _____
_____
_____
_____

15. Identify three organs of the lymphatic system:
_____
_____
_____

16. The branch of medicine that is concerned with the function of the heart and diseases affecting it is known as _____ .

17. Differentiate between an *embolism* and a *thrombus*. _____
_____
_____
_____

18. List three indications for performing an angiographic procedure for diagnostic purposes. _____
_____
_____

19. _____ are medications administered therapeutically to dissolve an arterial blood clot that has occluded a blood vessel.

20. What is the purpose of inserting a vena cava filter into the inferior vena cava? _____
_____
_____
_____

21. What is *embolization therapy?* _____
_____
_____
_____

22. Name three common embolization agents. _____
_____
_____
_____

23. What is the function of a *stent?* _____
_____

24. Describe the procedure for placing a stent in a blood vessel. _____
_____
_____
_____

25. What information should be included in an Informed Consent document for an angiographic procedure? _____
_____
_____
_____

26. What is the patient preparation for an angiogram with regard to food and drink? _____
_____

27. What is the most common site used to access an artery for an angiographic procedure? _____
_____

28. The method used to access the artery for an angiographic procedure is known as the _____ .

29. What is the purpose of applying pressure to the access site of the artery at the completion of the procedure? _____
_____

30. Following an angiogram, the patient stays in the hospital for careful observation for a period of up to _____ hours.

31. What is the function of a catheter? What is the advantage of using a catheter for an angiographic procedure? _____
_____
_____
_____

32. What is the purpose of the different end tips of the catheters? _____
_____

33. What type of contrast medium is used in angiography?
_____

34. Explain the need for a shifting (stepping) tabletop for a femoral angiogram. _____
_____
_____

35. Why is a guide wire used with a catheter? _____
_____
_____

36. Why is contrast medium administered with the use of a pressure injector as opposed to hand injection for angiography? _____
_____
_____
_____

37. A procedure known as _____
uses a computer to enhance the radiographic image by taking out unnecessary structures (ie, bones) and leaving the vessels filled with contrast medium.

38. The _____ valve is located between the right atrium and ventricle, whereas the _____
_____ valve is located between the left atrium and ventricle of the heart.

39. The left coronary artery divides into two branches: the _____ , which runs along the front border of the heart to the apex, and the _____
_____ , which passes along the back side of the heart toward the inferior wall.

40. Valvular disease is a/an _____ (contraindication/indication) for performing cardiac catheterization.

41. In a procedure known as _____ ,
a balloon catheter is placed in the coronary artery at the site of a lesion. The balloon is inflated, pushing the lesion against the arterial wall and restoring patency to the vessel.

42. Name two procedures that use a cutting device on a catheter to cut or shave away a lesion in an artery. _____
_____
_____

43. Identify the four main blood vessels that supply blood to the head. _____
_____
_____
_____

44. Arising from the left ventricle, the aorta begins at the aortic valve of the heart and continues to the approximate level of the _____ vertebra.

45. The celiac axis arises from the ventral surface of the abdominal aorta and branches into the following three arteries: _____
_____
_____

46. The superior mesenteric artery supplies blood to what area of the abdomen? _____
_____
_____

47. A 37-year-old male was scheduled for a renal angiogram. According to his history, he was not having any problems but was donating his left kidney to his sister, who had polycystic kidney disease. Why would a renal angiogram be performed in such a case? _____
_____
_____
_____

48. When performing a pulmonary angiogram, the femoral vein is usually accessed for insertion of the catheter. Trace the path that the radiologist would follow in guiding the catheter from the femoral vein to the left pulmonary artery. _____

_____

_____

_____

49. A lymphangiogram was ordered on a patient who had a history of unexplained peripheral swelling. Why was this exam ordered given the patient's history? _____

_____

_____

_____

50. When performing lymphangiography, why is a blue indicator dye injected into the webbing between the toes prior to the injection of contrast medium? Why is a radiograph taken 24 hours after the completion of the injection? ____

_____

_____

_____

_____

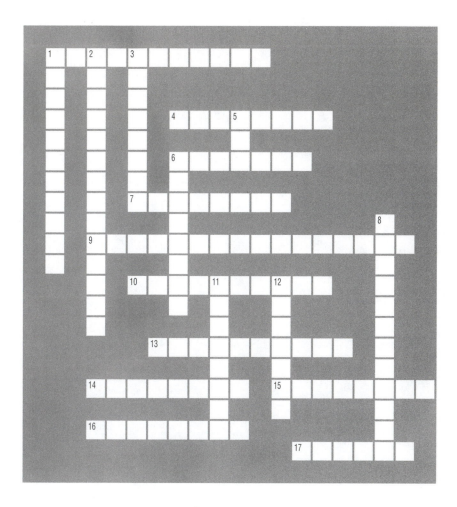

ACROSS

1. Communication between two vessels, such as the circle of Willis
4. Accumulation of clotted blood that leaks out of a blood vessel as the result of an injury
6. Malformation or absence of anatomic structures
7. Constriction or narrowing of a body opening, passage, or vessel
9. Hardening of the arteries
10. Longitudinal tearing of the intima of the aorta
13. Radiographic examination of the venous system within a specific region of the body following the injection of contrast medium
14. Insufficient blood supply to an organ or structure as a result of an obstruction in a blood vessel
15. Delivers contrast medium to the specific area of interest
16. Tumor in the lymphatic system that is usually malignant
17. Chest pain that is usually due to myocardial ischemia

DOWN

1. Incision of an artery
2. Radiographic examination of an artery or arteries in a specific region of the body following the administration of contrast medium
3. Blood clot that may partially or completely occlude the blood vessel
5. Arteriovenous malformation
6. Weak area in a vessel's wall causing it to balloon outward
8. Arrhythmic condition in which the muscles of the heart quiver and contract involuntarily
11. Blood clot or other foreign material that moves away from its site of formation and suddenly occludes an artery
12. Area of necrosed tissue due to a lack of blood supply

► CASE STUDY

1. A hearing-impaired patient is scheduled for a cardiac catheterization procedure. He is extremely anxious about having the procedure performed.

   ► Discuss the method you will use to explain the procedure to him.

   ► Do you envision any difficulties that might occur during the procedure as a result of the patient's hearing impairment?